CARDIOVASCULAR SURGERY

The HANDBOOKS *of* OPERATIVE SURGERY

THE STOMACH AND DUODENUM (4th ed.)

CLAUDE E. WELCH, M.D.

Visiting Surgeon, Massachusetts General Hospital
Clinical Professor of Surgery, Harvard Medical School

SURGICAL GYNECOLOGY (4th ed.)

J. P. GREENHILL, M.D.

Professor of Gynecology, Cook County Graduate School of Medicine
Senior Attending Obstetrician and Gynecologist, Michael Reese Hospital
Attending Gynecologist, Cook County Hospital

THE CHEST (4th ed.)

JULIAN JOHNSON, M.D., D.Sc. (Med)

Professor of Surgery, School of Medicine, University of Pennsylvania

HORACE MacVAUGH, III, M.D.

Assistant Professor of Clinical Surgery, School of Medicine, University of Pennsylvania

JOHN A. WALDHAUSEN, M.D.

Professor of Surgery and Chairman, Department of Surgery,
Milton S. Hershey School of Medicine, Pennsylvania State University

THE BILIARY TRACT, PANCREAS AND SPLEEN (4th ed.)

CHARLES B. PUESTOW, M.D.

Clinical Professor of Surgery, The Abraham Lincoln School of Medicine and
Graduate College, University of Illinois

SURGICAL UROLOGY (3d ed.)

R. H. FLOCKS, M.D.

Professor and Head, Department of Urology

DAVID CULP, M.D.

Professor of Urology, University of Iowa College of Medicine

THE HEAD AND NECK (3d ed.)

ROBERT A. WISE, M.D.
Clinical Professor of Surgery

HARVEY W. BAKER, M.D.
Associate Clinical Professor of Surgery, University of Oregon Medical School

---

CARDIOVASCULAR SURGERY (2d ed.)

ORMAND C. JULIAN, M.D., PH.D.
Professor of Surgery

WILLIAM S. DYE, M.D.
Clinical Professor of Surgery

HUSHANG JAVID, M.D., PH.D.
Professor of Surgery

JAMES A. HUNTER, M.D.
Associate Professor of Surgery

HASSAN NAJAFI, M.D.
Associate Professor of Surgery, The Abraham Lincoln School of Medicine, University of Illinois

---

SURGERY OF THE BREAST

HARRY W. SOUTHWICK, M.D.
Clinical Professor of Surgery, The Abraham Lincoln School of Medicine, University of Illinois

DANELY P. SLAUGHTER, M.D. (Deceased)
Clinical Professor of Surgery, The Abraham Lincoln School of Medicine, University of Illinois

LOREN J. HUMPHREY, M.D.
Associate Professor of Surgery, Emory University School of Medicine

---

REPAIR OF HERNIAS

MARK M. RAVITCH, M.D.
Professor of Surgery, University of Pittsburgh School of Medicine, and Surgeon-in-Chief, Montefiore Hospital, Pittsburgh

A HANDBOOK OF OPERATIVE SURGERY

CARDIOVASCULAR SURGERY

ORMAND C. JULIAN, M.D., Ph.D.

*Professor of Surgery, The Abraham Lincoln School of Medicine, University of Illinois;
Attending Surgeon, Rush-Presbyterian-St. Luke's Hospital, Chicago*

WILLIAM S. DYE, M.D.

*Clinical Professor of Surgery, The Abraham Lincoln School of Medicine, University of Illinois;
Attending Surgeon, Rush-Presbyterian-St. Luke's Hospital, Chicago*

HUSHANG JAVID, M.D., Ph.D.

*Professor of Surgery, The Abraham Lincoln School of Medicine, University of Illinois;
Rush-Presbyterian-St. Luke's Hospital, Chicago*

JAMES A. HUNTER, M.D.

*Associate Professor of Surgery, The Abraham Lincoln School of Medicine, University of Illinois;
Rush-Presbyterian-St. Luke's Hospital, Chicago*

HASSAN NAJAFI, M.D., M.S.

*Associate Professor of Surgery, The Abraham Lincoln School of Medicine, University of Illinois;
Attending Surgeon, Rush-Presbyterian-St. Luke's Hospital, Chicago*

SECOND EDITION

Illustrated by DIANE L. NELSON *and* RUSSELL CARLSON

YEAR BOOK MEDICAL PUBLISHERS • INC.

35 EAST WACKER DRIVE · CHICAGO

Second Edition, December 1970

Library of Congress Catalog Card Number: 78-119579

International Standard Book Number: 0-8151-4932-8

Dedicated to
OUR WIVES

Preface

THIS HANDBOOK is designed to be informative of the scope of
cardiovascular surgery. It deals almost exclusively with the technical aspects of the operative procedures which are used to restore
circulatory function in disease states and to correct congenital
anomalies. Despite its technical nature, it is primarily intended for
physicians with general interest in medicine and for general surgeons who will find here an account of the treatment possibilities
in a variety of conditions. Without such graphic portrayal as that
permitted by an operative handbook, some of these procedures may
remain obscure to those not directly engaged in the field, with the
result that patients may be denied useful treatment. It is not likely
that cardiovascular surgeons will benefit from this volume beyond
observing the individual technical maneuvers employed by the
authors in carrying out the procedures described.

Some liberties have been taken in exceeding the limitations of a
technical handbook by discussing examination and clinical diagnosis. However, the actual indications for the operations and
reviews of known results of the individual procedures are not considered. It is evident that a meaningful presentation of information
upon which a mature judgment in the application of surgery of this
type could be developed would require many volumes. Selection of
patients is generally left to those whose specialized experience in
the field has qualified them for the task. In many instances the final
evaluation of results of a procedure is far from being attained. The
inclusion of a procedure in this handbook is, therefore, not intended
to indicate that it is firmly established as an accepted operation
which will surely stand the test of the future.

The efforts of a great number of surgeons are represented in the surgical procedures included here. It is perhaps fortunate that bibliographic references to the reports which contributed to the development of the operations were not planned. Although many definite breakthroughs characterize the advance in the field, much of the progress has evolved through parallel work at several centers. We acknowledge the lack of identification of those who had most to do with the development of these operations, a defect overcome only in the few instances in which a surgeon's name has been applied by common usage.

We are grateful to our medical illustrators, Miss Diane L. Nelson, Mr. Russell Carlson and his assistant, Mrs. Ruth Best, and to Miss Gerry Stearns and our secretaries. We acknowledge with thanks the patient work of Mr. James L. Holman in organizing the process of completion of the volume.

ORMAND C. JULIAN
WILLIAM S. DYE
HUSHANG JAVID
JAMES A. HUNTER
HASSAN NAJAFI

Table of Contents

Section III. THE HEART and GREAT VESSELS

List of Illustrations

15

The Arterial System

CHAPTER 1

Introduction

THE SURGERY of the arterial system has as its objective re-establishment of the circulation to restore or to maintain normal function in tissues in which the blood supply has been impeded or threatened by the vascular lesion. The purely technical aspects of the problems in arterial surgery have long been overcome. Major advances in the application of these technics occurred when the understanding of the management and anesthesia problems in general surgery of comparable magnitude reached a suitable level. Further extension of the scope of arterial surgery to include progressively more major problems has been, and continues to be, a steady process.

Direct arterial surgery deals with arterial trauma, acute and chronic arterial obstruction and aneurysm. Reconstruction has been carried out with complete success in the arterial channels supplying most of the parts and organ systems of the body. There are distinct limitations in relation to its application to each variety of arterial lesion. Arterial surgery in trauma is perhaps the least limited, being influenced principally by the general severity of the patient's injury and the factor of time. In acute arterial occlusion, time is of primary importance in occlusions secondary to an embolus. The extent of the underlying pathology limits the success of treatment of an acute thrombosis superimposed on pre-existing arterial disease. The degree of success in dealing with chronic arterial occlusion depends on the extent of the disease and the size of the vessel involved. Consequently, the lesions most successfully treated are the localized arteriosclerotic changes involving major vessels. The less clearly defined processes of thromboangiitis obliterans and endarteritis obliterans, involving as they do the medium and small-sized vessels, are not approached by direct means. The progressive and dangerous course followed by aneurysms renders repair essential in most patients even though the magnitude of the surgical problem will be considerable in some.

Two major types of arterial reconstruction are available for restoration of circulation in most locations. These are (1) thromboendarterectomy, used in treatment of arteriosclerotic obstructions, and (2) grafts, used to restore circulation after removal of an arterial lesion or to by-pass an area of arterial occlusion. In many instances the indication for one of these technics as compared to the other may not be distinct.

The general evaluation of a patient with arterial disease extends beyond delineation of the local problem. An individual who has a symptom-producing arterial lesion in one area is often found to have significant but not yet symptomatic lesions in other locations, sometimes of more importance than the primary trouble. This is particularly true in the patient with arteriosclerosis. A significant proportion of patients with aortoiliac or femoral arteriosclerosis producing symptoms and signs of ischemia will, on complete evaluation, show renovascular, coronary or cerebral vascular disease. The most frequent serious complication of arterial surgery arises from an acute arterial occlusion in another area. The arteriosclerotic patient, therefore, is examined in relation to his renal function, and with particular attention if he is hypertensive. The coronary circulation is evaluated, and careful attention is given to eliciting a history of symptoms which might be attributed to intermittent cerebral ischemia.

Any other vascular lesion that is discovered must be evaluated as a possible contraindication to surgery. Also, it must be considered that this second area of vascular disease may be amenable to and require restoration. In the not uncommon case in which a significant carotid artery lesion is discovered in patients under consideration for other surgery, the prior removal of the carotid obstruction should be given serious thought.

CHAPTER 2

Clinical Evaluation

Vascular Examination

A PRACTICAL EVALUATION of the arterial system can be made very quickly and should be an integral part of the physical examination of every patient. It consists of palpation of the pulses in the extremities, neck and abdomen and observation of the character of the walls of palpable vessels. Auscultation provides information when sounds are made by the flow of blood through various arteries. Results of these observations should be recorded as habitually as are other routine parts of the examination. Normal observations positively recorded can be of great future value to the patient.

Arteries are palpated to determine not only the presence of pulses and the comparative strength on the two sides, but also the character of the arterial wall. This is particularly important, for example, in the region of the bifurcation of the common carotid artery, where an atherosclerotic lesion often produces a firm widening.

In the upper extremity the brachial and radial artery pulses are palpable, the ulnar pulse sometimes being difficult to feel. In the lower extremities the femoral artery particularly offers itself for easy palpation as to its size and the character of its wall (A). The popliteal space (B) is palpated using the fingers of both hands. The dorsalis pedis artery (C) is occasionally absent as a congenital variant. The posterior tibial artery pulse, palpable behind the medial malleolus (D), has not been observed to be congenitally displaced or absent.

The oscillometric reading (E) is of value in comparing the two extremities of the same individual and in determining the point along an extremity at which the artery is occluded.

PLATE 1

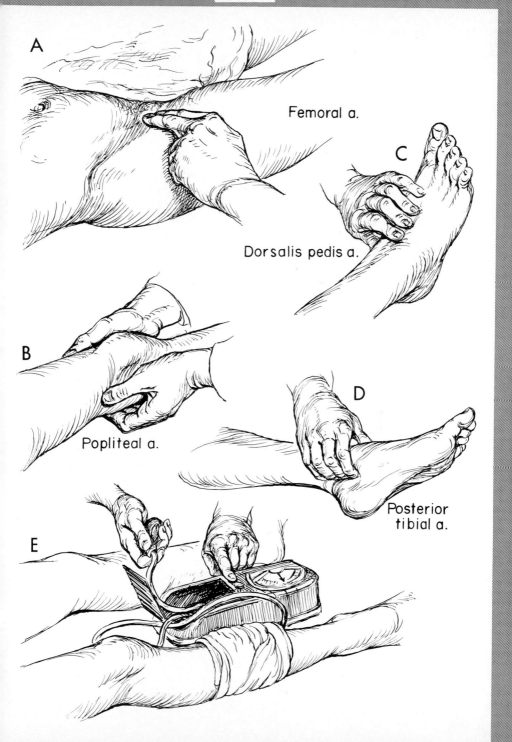

A — Femoral a.

B — Popliteal a.

C — Dorsalis pedis a.

D — Posterior tibial a.

E

The smooth lamellar flow of blood through the major arteries normally is quiet. Noises over the course of a vessel are usually indicative of some form of pathology. The causes of noises over blood vessels include (1) an abnormality of the pulse curve, such as that produced by aortic valvular insufficiency, (2) a communication between artery and vein, as in traumatic or congenital arteriovenous fistula and (3) stenosis or compression of a vessel producing turbulence of flow.

The commonest abrupt change in caliber of a vessel occurs in the *presence of an atherosclerotic* plaque producing stenosis. Distal to such an area of stenosis a systolic bruit is usually audible, and bruit is often the earliest sign of arterial disease. This sign may be present before there is any detectable diminution in the amplitude of the pulse or any change in its character compared to the alternate side.

The various locations in which bruit is audible are shown in Plate 2. Bruit at the carotid artery bifurcation is of great importance in the diagnosis of internal carotid artery stenosis and is most significant if a bruit is not present also over the common carotid artery on the same side. Bruits of vascular origin over the common carotid artery must be differentiated from a transmitted murmur of stenosis of the aortic valve. Abnormal systolic sounds over the subclavian artery may be heard in relation to either the supra- or infraclavicular course of the artery. They are sometimes affected by changes in position of the head, neck or shoulder. An instance of the inconstant presence of a bruit over the subclavian artery is observed in scalenus anticus syndrome, when the bruit appears as compression of the subclavian artery between the muscle and the first rib is developed in the rotated position of the head and neck.

The epigastric bruit may be a normal finding, but bruits over the abdomen in the hypochondriac regions on either side suggest stenosis of the renal artery or abnormalities of the splenic artery. Bruits over the aortic bifurcation are usually transmitted into the iliac fossa and into the femoral triangle.

PLATE 2

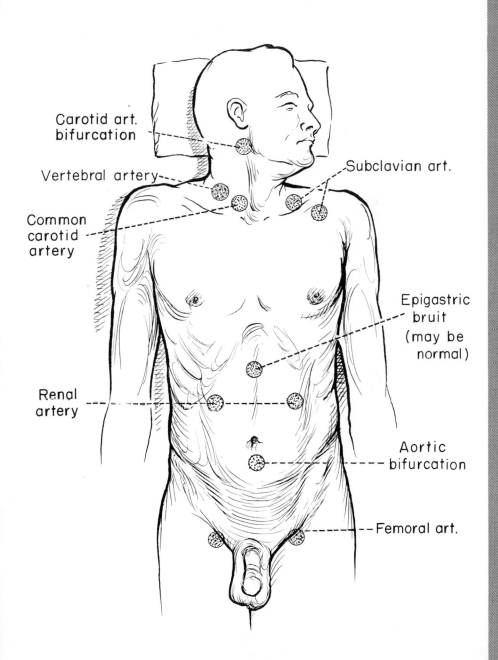

Carotid art.
bifurcation

Vertebral artery

Common
carotid
artery

Subclavian art.

Epigastric
bruit
(may be
normal)

Renal
artery

Aortic
bifurcation

Femoral art.

The production of a temporary sympathetic paralysis of the lower extremities through injection of local anesthetic agent into the region of the lumbar sympathetic ganglia is of value in the treatment of acute arterial spasm and in differentiating reflex arterial constriction from anatomic occlusion of the vessel. Careful evaluation of the effect of a sympathetic block aids in predicting the probable effect of surgical sympathectomy.

The patient is placed on his left side for the right lumbar block (*A*). By palpation of the bony landmarks, the levels of the transverse processes of the first, second and third lumbar vertebrae are approximated and may be marked. The point of needle introduction varies in its distance from the midline in proportion to the obesity of the patient, as is suggested in the cross-section diagram (*B*), in which the skin level of an obese patient is indicated by the dotted line. An 18 gauge, 6 1/2 – 7 in. needle is introduced through a procaine wheal and advanced obliquely downward (*a*) in a plane which is judged to reach the midline of the trunk an inch or two in front of the anterior surface of the vertebral bodies. The needle will most often meet bony obstruction at a depth of 1 1/2 – 2 1/2 in. as it reaches the transverse process. The needle is then withdrawn and redirected above or below the transverse process. The new direction (*b*) is selected at an angle more acute with the midline plane of the patient and strikes another bony obstruction as it reaches the side of the vertebral body. Redirection, elevating the tip of the needle away from the vertebral body, results in its free passage forward. It is advanced 1/2 to 3/4 in., so that the tip will lie someplace in the angle formed by the vertebral body, the psoas muscle and the vena cava (or the aorta on the left side of the patient). Needle introduction and injection is often done at three levels. Five to 10 ml. of local anesthetic solution is placed at each level.

PLATE 3

A

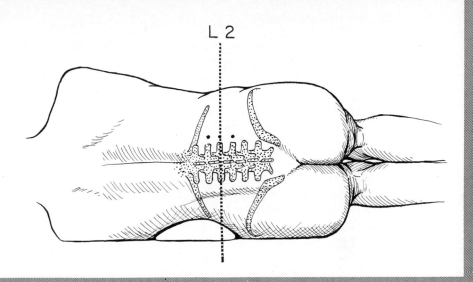

L 2

B

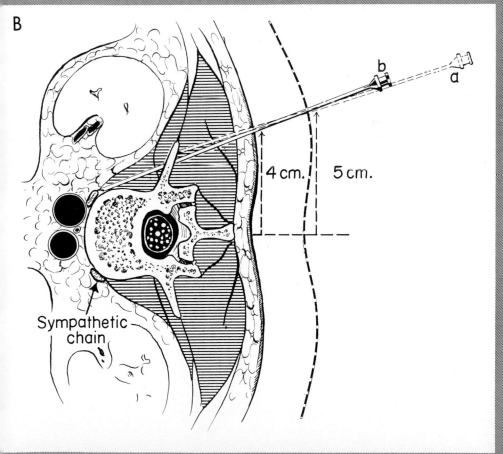

b

a

4 cm.   5 cm.

Sympathetic
chain

Injection of an anesthetic solution into the region of the inferior cervical and first dorsal ganglia produces an anatomically incomplete, but functionally very effective, interruption of the sympathetic innervation of the upper extremity and the head. The anterior route of injection, because of its simplicity, is commonly used for temporary sympathetic denervation of the upper extremity, in spite of the fact that some sympathetic fibers contributing to the brachial plexus are not interrupted. Sympathetic block in this region helps to differentiate between arterial spasm and anatomic arterial occlusion in the upper extremity. It relieves pain of sympathetic origin in the arm. There is also convincing clinical evidence that it increases cerebral circulation under certain conditions.

The injection is done with the patient lying on his back and is made more convenient if the chin is elevated by extending the neck (*A*), though this is not necessary. A procaine wheal is produced just above the clavicle over the medial edge of the sternocleidomastoid muscle. The sternocleidomastoid muscle and the carotid vessels are moved laterally and the trachea and retrotracheal tissues, including the esophagus, are pushed medially by deep pressure between these structures with finger or thumb (*B*). The depression of the skin which results from this maneuver brings the anterior surface of the neck close to the cervical spine. This position is maintained throughout the injection. A 2 in., 22 gauge needle is then advanced through the wheal in a posterior, somewhat lateral direction until it touches a bony prominence which will be in the region of the transverse process of the first thoracic vertebra or the base of the first rib (*C*). The needle point is slightly withdrawn from contact with the bone and, after a trial aspiration, 5 – 10 ml. of the anesthetic solution is injected.

Evidence of a successful injection will be the development of Horner's sign. Usually the first evidence of change in the extremity is a dilatation of the veins of forearm, wrist and hand. Somewhat later the skin of the extremity and of the side of the face becomes dry and, unless severe arterial obstruction is present, perceptibly warmer.

PLATE 4

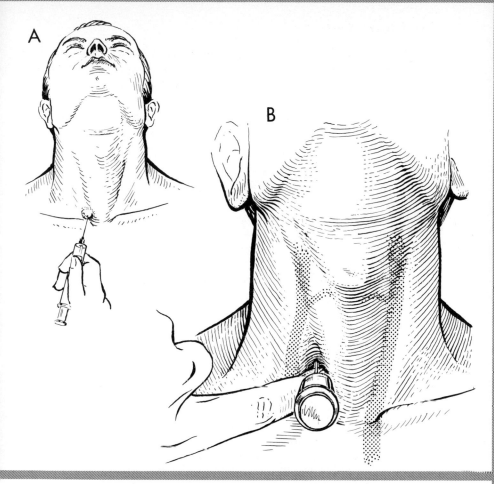

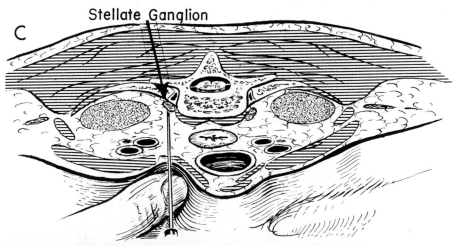

Stellate Ganglion

Visualization by x-ray of the lumens of various parts of the arterial system during the injection of a radiopaque solution provides the detailed information of disease involvement which is often required for accurate application of surgical treatment. The hazards of the procedure, both in general and in a specific patient, must be compared with the value of the information which will be obtained before these techniques are used.

The dangers of arteriography consist of damage to the vessel wall at the point of introduction of the contrast medium, the vasoconstrictor effect of the solution on the vessels through which it flows, and the possible damage to organs and structures supplied by the vessels being visualized or by arteries in the same region which will inadvertently carry the solution, although they themselves are not being directly visualized.

The local trauma produced depends on the amount of disease present in the vessel at the point of injection and on the skill of the operator. The greatest damage would be produced by elevation of an atherosclerotic plaque as the needle passes through the vessel wall, or by introducing a portion of the radiopaque solution into the vessel wall in the event that the end of the needle is not advanced entirely into the lumen.

Vasoconstriction of sufficient severity and duration to produce thrombosis of narrowed sclerotic arteries is a remote danger. A preliminary sympathetic block or the addition of procaine to the injected solution can diminish this hazard. The possibility that a parenchymatous organ, such as the kidney, may be damaged by abrupt perfusion with the substances used, even in the absence of arterial disease within the organ, is suggested by experimental and clinical evidence of disturbance of renal function after aortography. The contrast mediums currently available for arteriography vary in renal toxicity, and new compounds appear from time to time. Every advantage should be taken of selection of the solution and of its concentration, volume and rate of injection. It is essential that all hazards be taken into account in deciding whether or not to use arteriography in an individual patient. Careful evaluation of the physical findings, particularly in disease of the lower aorta and iliac systems, often provides sufficient information for the accurate application of reconstructive arterial surgery. In many instances, direct surgical exploration of the vessels distal to the area of maximum disease will provide more information with less risk to the patient.

The danger of x-ray exposure to the operator is a considerable factor. He must be protected not only by the usual lead apron but also by use of tubing connections from syringe to needle of sufficient length and a screen to shield his hands. A remote-control mechanical device for injection is valuable to avoid operator exposure as well as to provide rapid injection when desirable.

Misleading interpretations of arteriograms sometimes result from inadequate filling of the vessels, poor timing of the exposures in relation to the injection and, in arteriosclerosis, from the localization of the mural thickening to one aspect of the circumference of the vessel. Inadequate filling should immediately be recognized and the poor contrast film not be considered in diagnosis. If exposure is timed too early after injection, the film shows an apparent obstruction which actually represents the distal end of the advancing dye. A thick posterior or dorsal plaque in a vessel may go unnoticed if the *en face* ribbon-like lumen is wide. The only way to avoid this misinformation is to obtain roentgenograms in two planes.

Injection of contrast medium into the common femoral artery for visualization of the arteries of the leg is done either by percutaneous puncture of the artery or by injection under direct vision. Surgical exposure of the artery for injection is required if the vessel wall is markedly thickened, as determined by palpation, or if there is no femoral pulse due to aortoiliac obstruction.

An 18 gauge needle is of sufficient caliber for the rate of injection required in femoral artery visualization. The needle should have a short bevel so that the needle point will be less likely to damage the far wall of the vessel when the entire tip is within the vessel lumen. The site of puncture is just beneath the lower edge of Poupart's ligament where the common femoral artery is more firmly held by surrounding tissues. A procaine wheal is raised directly over the pulse just below Poupart's ligament (*A*). The arteriography needle is introduced through the wheal down on to the vessel. It is directed upward at not more than a 10–15 degree angle (*B*). The vessel is stabilized between two fingers. As the needle is advanced, the pulsation of the vessel will be palpated through it; with continued firm pressure it will penetrate the vessel wall.

A free return flow of blood through the needle, which persists as the needle is rotated on its long axis, indicates that the lumen has been fully entered. Connections are then made for injection, using lock-type fittings to syringe and needle and a generous segment of securely fastened plastic tubing which will not expand under pressure.

The volume of contrast medium injected rarely should exceed 20 ml. The rate of injection varies somewhat with the type of lesion being examined. In an occlusive lesion, such as that illustrated in *C* and *D*, a relatively slow rate of injection of the first half of the contrast medium will give time for visualization of the artery distal to the occlusion. If the rate is speeded up just before the x-ray exposure is made, the proximal artery will be more fully visualized. When done under local anesthesia, the patient must be warned that some burning pain will be experienced briefly and that he will be expected to avoid moving the extremity during this period.

PLATE 5

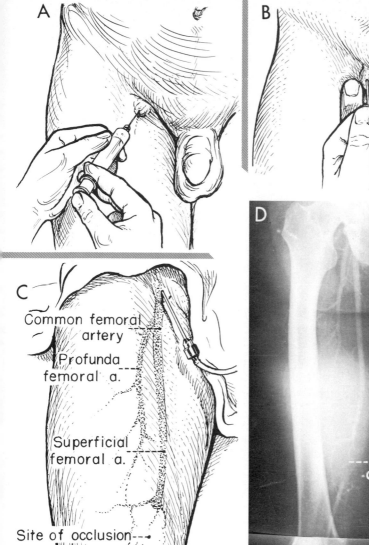

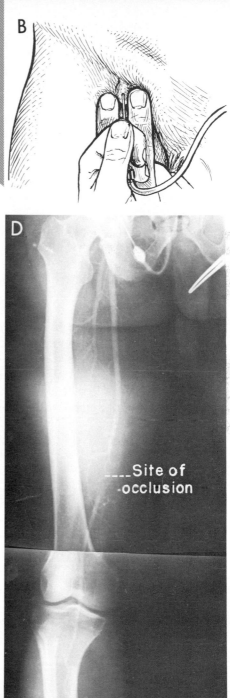

C

Common femoral artery

Profunda femoral a.

Superficial femoral a.

Site of occlusion

D

Site of occlusion

Translumbar aortography is a reliable method of visualizing the abdominal aorta and the iliac vessels. Although local anesthesia may suffice for the procedure, the best control is obtained through the use of a rapidly eliminated general anesthetic agent, a suitable muscular relaxant and endotracheal intubation. The patient lies prone on the x-ray table, suitably positioned over the cassette or film changer. An exposure is made to verify the patient's position and the x-ray exposure factors. While this film is being developed, the patient's back is prepared and draped. A 7 in., 17 gauge needle with a stylet is used for the injection. The needle is introduced just below the left twelfth rib, 2 1/2 – 3 in. lateral to the midline. The angle of introduction in relation to the longitudinal axis is approximately that which will direct the needle toward the right axilla (*A*). The angle with the transverse vertical body plane is about 15 degrees. Bony obstructions may be encountered at the levels of the transverse process and the vertebral body (*B*). The needle is gently withdrawn upon reaching such obstructions and is manipulated past the structure until it passes the vertebral body and is felt to enter the aorta after encountering its firm, pulsating wall. The stylet may be removed when the aortic pulse is felt through the needle. Connections are made through secure fastenings to a 30 cc. syringe by way of a plastic tube.

To obviate intramural injection of the dye, which is possibly the most damaging accident that may occur, 2 – 4 ml. of dye is injected and an x-ray exposure made. Accurate placement of the needle will be indicated if there is no visualization of contrast medium; an intramural injection or the inadvertent placement of the needle into a branch rather than into the aortic lumen will be shown on this test film.

Twenty to 30 ml. of contrast medium is then injected as rapidly as possible. The appropriate exposure is made near, but not at the end of the injection (inset).

PLATE 6

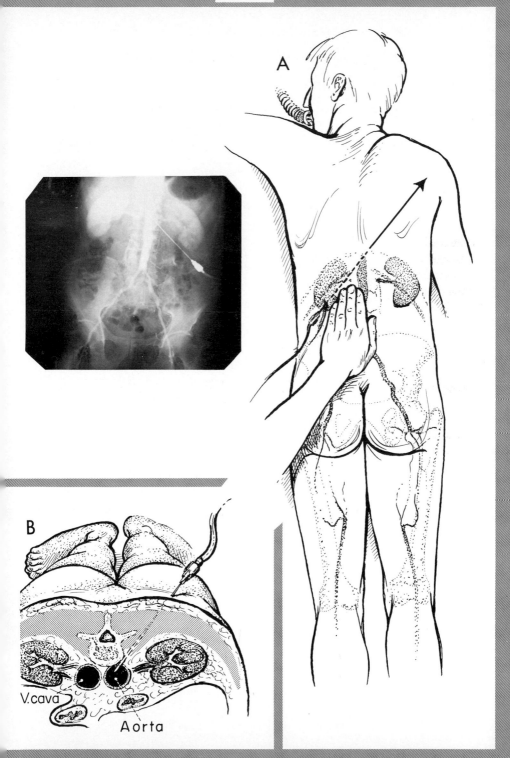

A

B

V.cava

Aorta

The ascending thoracic aorta is best opacified by contrast medium injected through a catheter advanced by one route or another to lie just above the valve. Various types of plastic and woven catheters may be used for this purpose. They are introduced either by percutaneous puncture of the right carotid or the femoral artery or through the femoral or brachial artery after its exposure under local anesthesia.

Percutaneous puncture of the carotid artery is permissible when this vessel itself is not abnormal. The use of one type of catheter-needle arrangement is illustrated in Plate 7. With the patient supine, the neck moderately extended and rotated to the left, a procaine wheal is made in the skin over the most proximal and easily palpable portion of the right common carotid artery (*A*). The needle-plastic catheter arrangement shown in *B* is made by passing the 18–20 gauge needle through the wall of the catheter at such a distance from its end that the needle protrudes beyond the catheter. A nick in the skin made with a scalpel will facilitate the passage of needle and catheter. The needle is introduced into the carotid artery in an obliquely downward direction (*C*). It is then carefully slipped out of the catheter, which is advanced downward into the ascending aorta (*D*). Fluoroscopic control is not essential, because the catheter can be advanced until aortic valve action is clearly felt. The catheter is then withdrawn 2 cm. to avoid loss of dye into the left ventricle. A mechanical injector is essential to minimize the amount of dye required and to intensify the contrast. The aortogram (*E*) reveals the lesion.

When the catheter is passed upward from the femoral artery, visualization under the fluoroscope is required to avoid entering the brachiocephalic branches. Some control of the advancing end of the catheter can be obtained as it passes around the aortic arch by setting it in a curved shape. The catheter is held straight during the initial progress up the aorta by a long wire stylet which is removed when the arch is reached.

PLATE 7

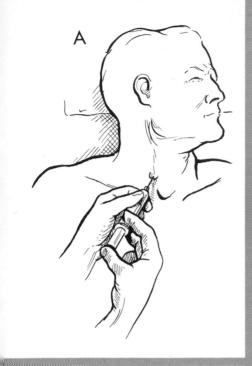

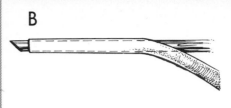

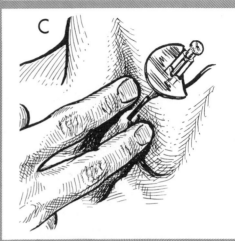

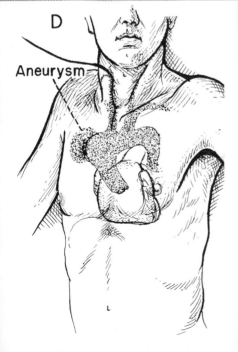

Aneurysm

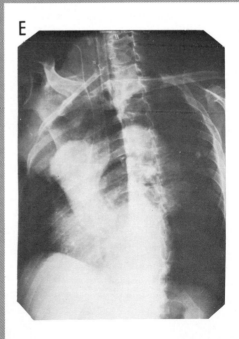

Satisfactory, but often not brilliant, visualization of the thoracic aorta and its brachiocephalic branches results from the very rapid injection of contrast medium through a catheter placed in the right atrium, the right ventricle or the pulmonary artery. The catheter is introduced through a limb vein (*A*) and is advanced to the desired central position (*B*).

The injecting syringe must be activated by a mechanical device to concentrate the bolus of dye. The material traverses the lesser circulation and returns to the left heart to be passed on to the aorta and its branches. A rapid film-changing device must be used to obtain satisfactory results.

This method is more informative in lesions of the arch, such as aneurysm (*C*), dissecting aneurysm or coarctation, than in those of the branches of the arch. The dilution of the dye which results from passage through the pulmonary circuit limits the value of the visualization of these smaller vessels. The distinct advantage of this route compared to retrograde catheterization of the ascending aorta is that it avoids the danger of passing the catheter through the thoracic aorta in the presence of a fragile lesion. The frequent accompaniment of lesions of the iliofemoral and abdominal aortic regions with degenerative disease of the thoracic aorta also limits the feasibility of passing a catheter in a retrograde manner from below.

PLATE 8

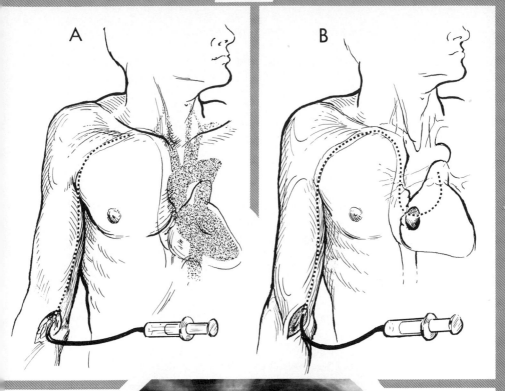

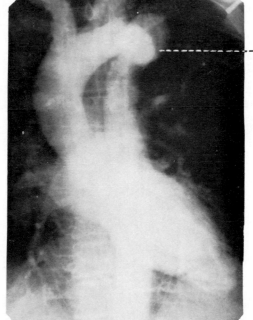

Aneurysm

The subclavian artery and its clinically most important branch, the vertebral artery, are visualized by direct puncture of the subclavian artery by way of a supraclavicular approach. However, they may be very adequately outlined in the more general arteriographic picture obtained by transvenous visualization of the thoracic arch or by the retrograde arch aortogram (Plates 7 and 8). If the catheter used for retrograde thoracic aortography is introduced through the brachial artery on the side in which subclavian and vertebral visualization is desired, an additional injection can be made when the catheter has been withdrawn from the aorta and its end lies in the subclavian artery.

Direct puncture of the subclavian artery is made at a point approximating the medial border of the scalenus anticus muscle. This method cannot be utilized unless the subclavian pulse is clearly palpable. The needle is directed through a procaine wheal (*A*) in a medial and downward direction, the needle being approximately in the plane of the clavicle, as shown in *B*. In this position, the point of contact with the vessel is less than 3 cm. in the oblique direction from the point of introduction through the skin. Great rapidity of injection is not required, and the clarity of visualization of the central portions of the artery can be enhanced by applying the blood pressure cuff high on the arm (*C*). The arteriogram reproduced in *D* shows the vertebral artery and other branches of the proximal subclavian artery and discloses an aneurysm of the third portion of the subclavian artery. In addition, the artery to the upper extremity is completely obstructed at the junction of the subclavian and axillary portions. The injection in this particular patient was made lateral to the scalenus anticus muscle, where the maximum pulsation was felt, because the fact was not appreciated that this increased pulsation was due to aneurysmal dilatation of the vessel.

PLATE 9

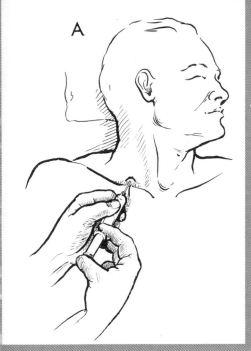

A

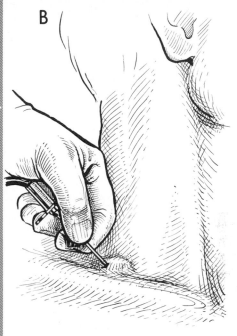

B

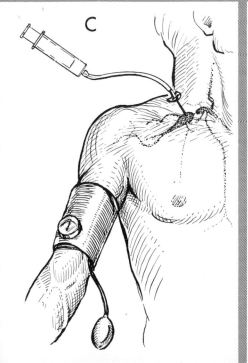

C

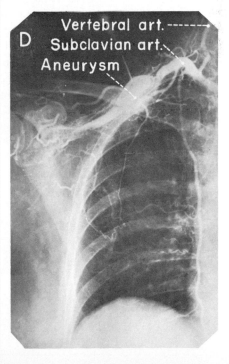

D

Vertebral art. --------
Subclavian art.
Aneurysm

CHAPTER 3

Arterial Injury

VARIOUS ELEMENTS of the environment of an arterial injury increase the difficulties in attaining the objective of its treatment, namely, the restoration of circulatory function. Frequently a vascular injury is just one of the important aspects of a compound injury, and the general destruction of tissues in the area makes difficult the task of isolation and control of vessels for their repair. When contamination is present, the surgeon is faced with the problem of implanting a blood vessel graft or prosthesis in a suboptimal field. A successful result under such circumstances attests to the thoroughness with which the wound was excised and otherwise cleansed. Further, the requirement that blood vessel injuries be repaired at the earliest possible time in order to prevent irreversible tissue changes places an unusual demand on availability of personnel and facilities equipped for specialized techniques. However, the same could be said of specialized orthopedic or neurosurgical techniques in treatment of a compound injury involving artery, nerve and bone, and the vascular problem need not be overwhelming if proper attention is given some fundamentals. Indeed, in handling a compound injury involving several systems, even the well-trained general surgeon may well be aware that an individual specially trained in the field might do better in dealing with each of the problems. This cannot affect his fulfillment of the demands of early and thorough reconstructive surgery.

Several factors are involved in a major vascular injury. These may be listed as follows: (1) hemorrhage and interruption of blood supply result from the arterial injury; (2) vein damage also causes blood loss and occlusion of the vessel, which in this case may produce important edema; (3) progressive thrombosis of the injured artery increases the occlusive effect of the lesion; (4) reflex constriction of the arteries of the entire region amplifies the effect of the traumatic obstruction.

Of these, the factors relating directly to the arterial injury, namely, hemorrhage and occlusion, have self-evident effects on the general surgical management. Hemorrhage from a venous injury has the same implications as that from the artery but is usually of lesser severity. Venous insufficiency is sometimes a major factor. It may be due entirely to damage to the vein, or it may be augmented by venous compression caused by accumulation of blood in tissues confined by fascial enclosures. Particularly in injuries about the elbow and knee, the immediate swelling and sometimes the further embarrassment of venous drainage produced by immobilization when bone is involved have serious consequences. Under such circumstances the forearm or leg can suffer ischemic damage which, within a few hours, brings about irreparable changes in the nerves and muscles. It is important to realize that this may occur, even without injury to an artery, simply on the basis of tissue pressure which inactivates the circulation through the vessels within the fascial enclosure.

Progressive thrombosis of the arterial lumen above and below the point of injury begins with the clot that forms in response to damage. The same phenomenon occurs after an embolic occlusion of an artery, but the use of anticoagulants which is usual in managing this problem in embolism cannot ordinarily be applied in trauma. This factor is important because it increases the urgent need of early repair and because it demands that the surgeon be particularly careful to clear the artery of clots distal to the injury at the time of repair. For this reason, in preparing the patient for repair of a damaged artery in an extremity, the entire part must be included in the surgical field. This is to permit exposure of the vessels at other locations distally for retrograde irrigation to remove thrombi or for arteriotomy for their direct removal.

General reflex vascular constriction in the area of an injury is an important feature of any arterial injury, but it is particularly prominent in injuries to the upper extremity where vasomotor control is most richly supplied. Some of this reflex activity can be combated by procaine infiltration of the appropriate portion of the sympathetic nervous system. Sympathetic block is often important, because the presence of diffuse vasospasm increases the difficulty of restoring circulation in the injured part after repair of the artery. These reflexes also serve in some instances to obscure the diagnosis. As will be noted later, many arterial injuries are not accompanied by external hemorrhage or development of an enclosed hematoma. In such a case the diagnosis of a traumatic occlusion of a major artery may be confused with a diminution in arterial supply attributable to reflex vasospasm. This differential diagnosis is aided by a sympathetic block, but there are certain leads in general evaluation that are helpful. The cutaneous pallor and the loss of pulses distal to the area of injury, which always occur in traumatic occlusion of major vessels, may be equaled by reflex vasospasm without actual arterial involvement, but the cyanosis which may accompany either situation is likely to be severe only in vascular spasm. Also, sensory loss and paralysis of small muscles in the distal part of the extremity follow arterial occlusion because of ischemia of peripheral nerves; they do not appear in response to vascular spasm. This is perhaps the most valued point of differentiation. However, it is entirely confused if there is a possibility that the trauma has also involved the nerve supply.

For success in treatment of an arterial injury, points which need particular attention begin with early diagnosis and appropriate repair. Then, during the reconstruction, there follows the need of the greatest possible attention to decontamination of the wound by debridement or excision, the development of the wound into a very adequate surgical exposure, the obtaining of proximal and distal control of the arterial injury, the removal of thrombi and, finally, nonconstrictive repair of the artery using a graft if needed.

It has already been mentioned that the venous elements in a vascular injury can assume importance if the extent of injury is sufficient to inhibit venous drainage of the part. If vein alone is injured, the resulting edema may be initiated immediately, whereas edema will occur only after arterial repair if both vein and artery were occluded. In either event the edema occasionally becomes so severe as to bring circulation to a standstill in the distal part of the extremity. Tense swelling of forearm or calf with progressive anesthesia of hand or foot and loss of pulse requires the same immediacy of treatment as does an arterial occlusion. Since veins are rarely subject to direct repair, the treatment consists in releasing the pressure in the swollen part by fasciotomy. Generous longitudinal incision of the deep fascia of leg or forearm accomplishes this. Whether or not the skin is repaired thereafter depends on the tension which might be required. Delay when this procedure is indicated will result in ischemic damage of nerves and muscle, leading to fibrosis, contraction and neurologic deficits. The familiar form of this result is Volkmann's ischemic contracture of the forearm.

Some arterial injuries do not interfere acutely with the blood supply of the involved part. These are pulsating hematoma, arteriovenous fistula and delayed post-traumatic true aneurysm, as well as a form of post-traumatic aneurysm seen in the thoracic aorta which seems to be a combination of elements of true aneurysm, pulsating hematoma and arterial contusion. If the principle of early repair of injured vessels is strictly followed, pulsating hematoma and arteriovenous fistula will rarely be allowed to become established lesions. True aneurysm, the result of traumatic weakening of the arterial wall with later stretching, is a rare but distinct lesion.

The most interesting of this group of nonoccluding arterial lesions is the traumatic thoracic aneurysm which has received much recent attention. It follows crushing trauma to the chest and is characteristically localized to the descending aorta just distal to the left subclavian artery. The resulting expanding lesion can be slow to develop and its discovery delayed. The fundamental lesion appears to be a tear, sometimes completely circumferential, in the intima and inner medial layers which allows the expansile force of blood pressure to be exerted on the remaining arterial wall. The possibility of such a lesion following chest injury suggests that x-ray examinations be done at intervals for some time after such trauma.

An injury to an artery of significant size takes precedence over most other lesions produced by trauma, with the outstanding exceptions of those which inhibit respiration and some head injuries. Injury to an artery is of primary importance because of occlusion of the injured artery with resulting ischemia and because of the loss of blood that results if the arterial injury communicates freely to the outside.

Injury to veins is not important so far as the circulation of a part is concerned except when there is extensive disruption of the major venous drainage of an extremity. This is encountered when an extensive, usually crushing, injury produces much swelling within the deep fascia which, added to direct damage to the veins, may cause such deficiency in venous drainage that the limb is imperiled.

Arterial injuries are produced by incised wounds or lacerations and by puncture wounds, all of these resulting in loss of blood either to the outside or into the tissues surrounding the injury. Another type of arterial injury—a contusion—is produced by a displaced fragment of a fracture or by the external application of a blunt force.

The injury illustrated in *A* is of the incised or lacerated type. The tendency of a cleanly incised wound of an artery to become deformed because of the longitudinal elasticity of the vessel is shown. This is the type of arterial trauma most likely to produce severe external bleeding, because the deforming elasticity of the vessel serves to keep the arterial wound open. If the vessel is actually transected the bleeding is less, because the ends retract and constrict, affording a better opportunity for thrombus formation.

The traumatic lesion illustrated in *B* is one produced by the posterior displacement of a supracondylar femoral fracture. *C* shows how trauma to the arm is incurred by catching the weight of the body (perhaps in a fall) on the inner aspect of the arm. Also shown is the typical bumper injury which may produce contusion of the popliteal artery. The resultant lesion is termed a contusion or intramural hematoma; it is shown in longitudinal section in *C*. The blood flow through the injured vessel is obstructed by the hemorrhage and by the swelling which develops in the wall of the vessel. External loss of blood does not occur.

PLATE 10

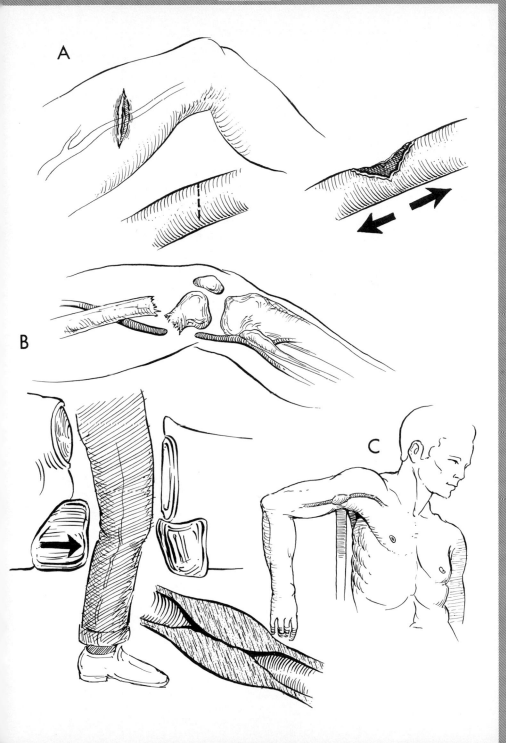

The intramural hematoma or contusion of a blood vessel is of singular importance because its presence may not be appreciated due to the lack of signs of arterial trauma such as hemorrhage into the tissues with formation of a palpable hematoma or external bleeding. The diagnosis depends on recognizing the presence of an arterial occlusion. Differentiation between a true injury of the artery with interruption of blood flow and an apparent cessation of blood flow because of intense vasoconstriction frequently requires use of a sympathetic ganglion block; only rarely is an arteriogram necessary. A period of observation will usually resolve the indecision, but it is probably better to explore an artery suspected of injury and find it uninjured than to miss the fact that the arterial circulation was interrupted.

Plate 11 illustrates the surgical repair of a contusion of the brachial artery incurred by a forceful compression in this area. The incision over the brachial artery is shown in *A*. The exploration, which in this region is done under local anesthesia, is illustrated in *B*. The adequacy of the exposure is important, as is the identification of the important nerves for their preservation and inspection for injury.

In this lesion the external evidence of injury to the blood vessel may be of a lesser extent than the actual damage to its walls. The exposure allows for adequate removal of vessel beyond the extent of obvious injury (*C*). The longitudinal and transverse sections shown in *D* and *E* indicate that the lumen of the vessel is compressed and obliterated by swelling and hemorrhage within the coats of the vessel; a propagating thrombus is seen to be forming at both the proximal and distal ends of the area of injury.

[Reconstruction of contused artery *continued on page 50.*]

PLATE 11

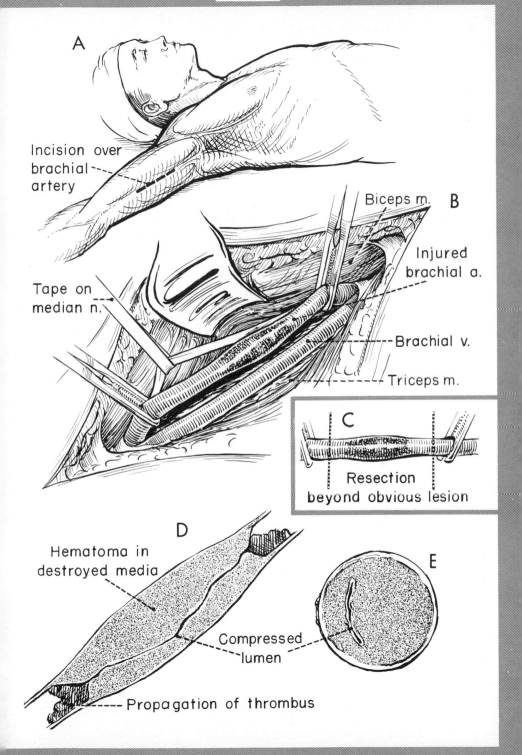

A

Incision over brachial artery

B

Biceps m.

Injured brachial a.

Tape on median n.

Brachial v.

Triceps m.

C

Resection beyond obvious lesion

D

Hematoma in destroyed media

E

Compressed lumen

Propagation of thrombus

The region of the intramural hematoma is shown in *F* in somewhat more detail, disclosing the disruption of the media and elastica of the vessel. The levels of transection of the vessel are again indicated. It should be emphasized that if transection is done first through an area which proves to be injured, more vessel should be excised. The line of transection may be at right angles to the longitudinal axis of the vessel or, as shown here, placed at a somewhat oblique angle.

G illustrates two fundamentals of repair at this stage. Clots which may have formed proximal to the point of injury are flushed out by the forceful flow of blood from above, and the distal propagating thrombus, if one has formed, is removed by aspiration until a good return flow of blood is obtained. Heparin diluted in saline is ordinarily injected distalward to prevent re-formation of soft clots.

Restoration of continuity of the artery by direct suture can almost never be performed after removal of a contused section of vessel. In this instance a vein graft is used to replace the resected contused artery. Autogenous saphenous vein grafts are used, with the graft positioned to allow proper flow through the valves (Plate 14). A Dacron prosthesis may be used if the vein graft is not available. The interposed vein graft is shown in *H*.

PLATE 11

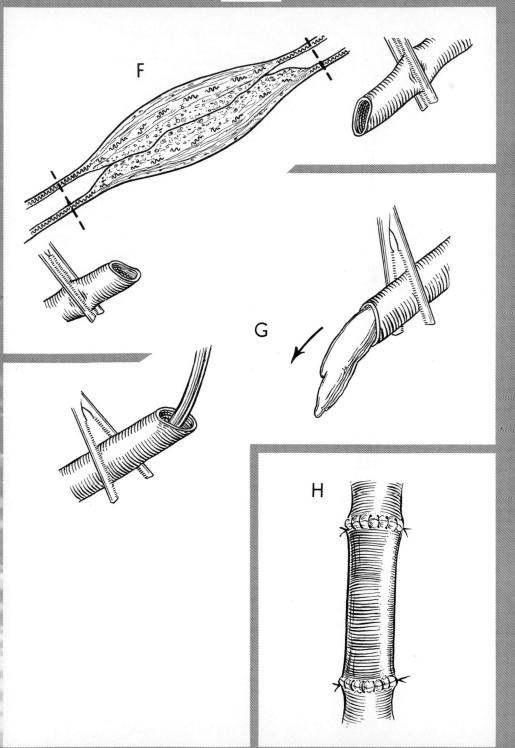

The management of a lacerated wound from which there is free hemorrhage, either arterial or venous, involves the steps illustrated in Plate 12.

In *A*, debridement of the wound is started. Proximal control of the artery may be obtained through a separate incision, if needed. Before preparation of the extremity, manual compression or a local pressure dressing may be used to control bleeding. Tourniquets are rarely used but may be in place at the time of the patient's admission to the hospital.

During repair of a lacerated artery, it is sometimes necessary to expose far distal branches of the vessel for retrograde removal of clots. Therefore, the entire extremity should be prepared and draped. Less elaborate preparation might consist simply of surgical preparation of the skin down to the tips of the toes and covering of the distal part of the extremity with drapes until it becomes evident that an incision at the popliteal or ankle level is necessary.

Preparation of the area of the wound consists, first, of thorough cleaning of the skin away from the wound. During this cleansing, the wound is kept covered with sterile gauze to prevent washing of contamination into the area. Then, with the surrounding area cleansed, the wound edges are prepared and the drape applied. When there is active bleeding, use of the tourniquet or manual compression is continued until the wound has been excised and lengthened for adequate exposure and the artery controlled within the confines of the wound.

The wide exposure illustrated in *B* is essential for restoration of circulation, which is the aim of the operation. The artery is shown isolated proximally and distally and lifted with tapes in preparation for the application of some type of atraumatic arterial forceps. In the drawing the vein is shown to be contused and not actively bleeding.

In *C*, the artery and vein are shown following reconstruction by end-to-end anastomosis, which is detailed in Plate 13. More often the injured vein is simply ligated. Reconstruction of the artery frequently requires a graft. The technique of implanting a vein graft is shown in Plate 14.

PLATE 12

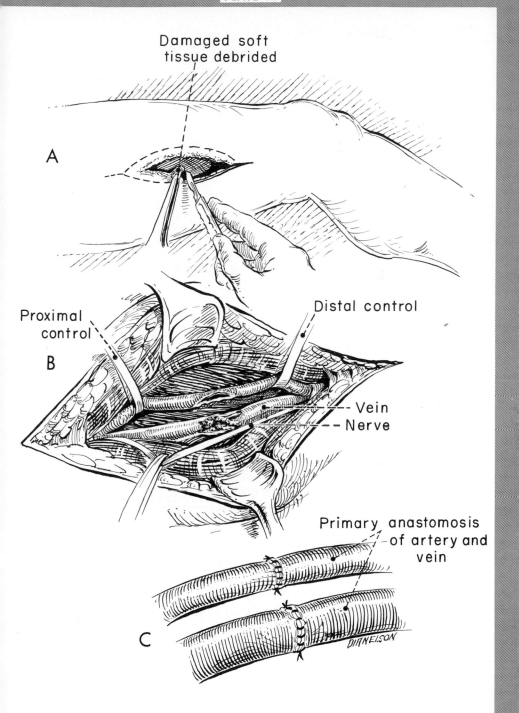

A — Damaged soft tissue debrided

B — Proximal control — Distal control — Vein — Nerve

C — Primary anastomosis of artery and vein

DIRNELSON

Repair of the artery itself is carried out in one of several ways. In a very clean wound, without devitalized tissue, some form of direct repair may be done. Direct repair cannot be depended upon if there is severe contamination or if the artery or the surrounding tissues are crushed.

A sharply incised stab wound, partially or completely transecting the artery, is illustrated in *A*. The vein which was either incised or torn has been ligated, and proximal and distal control of the artery has been obtained. The deformity of the artery produced by its elasticity is reduced by traction on the two arterial clamps. In this figure, which represents, unfortunately, a rare situation, the linear character of the arterial wound is evident as soon as retraction is overcome, and the wound is simply repaired (*B* and *C*) with an over-and-over suture using fine arterial silk.

In *D* the more usual, irregular laceration of the artery is illustrated, again after ligation of the accompanying vein and the placing of controlling clamps above and below the lesion. The damaged segment is being removed in *E*. The use of vein grafts or of arterial prostheses diminishes the absolute importance of direct repair, and therefore the principle of removal of all damaged vessel rather than the avoidance of the need for a graft is of maximum importance.

Approximation of the vessel ends (*F*) is obtained by traction on the arterial forceps, and a circumferential suture line composing the anastomosis is started at two points on the vessel (*G*). In a normal vessel, the sutures are placed 1–3 mm. from the edge of the vessel and 1–2 mm. apart. A simple over-and-over suture (*H*) is routinely applied. Great care is exercised to prevent pursestringing of the suture. It is tied after completing one-half the anastomosis, and the vessel is turned over (*I*) to bring the second half of the anastomosis into view.

PLATE 13

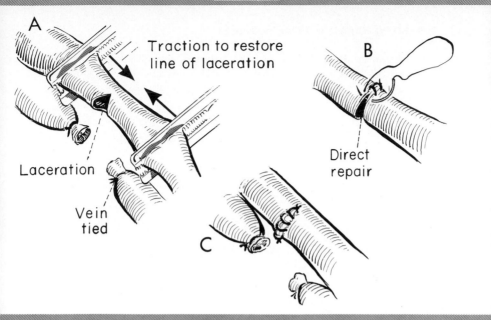

A

Traction to restore
line of laceration

B

Laceration

Direct
repair

Vein
tied

C

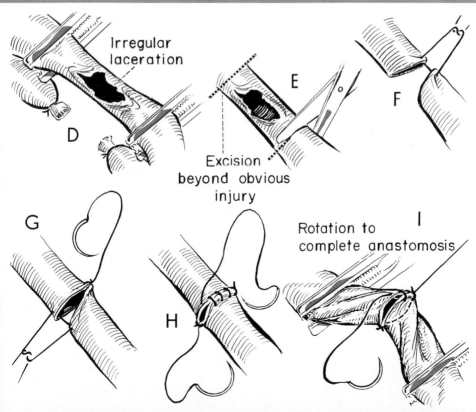

Irregular
laceration

D

E

F

Excision
beyond obvious
injury

G

Rotation to
complete anastomosis

I

H

The adequacy of removal of damaged artery must not be compromised in an attempt to preserve enough vessel length for direct anastomosis. To do so will result in leaving behind damaged vessel which may be the source of obstruction due to edema, prolonged spasm of the segment, increasing intramural hematoma or the production of an anastomosis under too great longitudinal tension.

Either an autogenous vein graft or an arterial prosthesis may be used to avoid these difficulties. A segment of vein for autogenous graft may be taken from the long saphenous, the external jugular or the superficial femoral vein. The adventitia is completely removed to facilitate passage of sutures. The graft is placed in such a way that the valves will not obstruct the flow of arterial blood (*A*). The proximal anastomosis is made first (*B*), using a continuous over-and-over suture of fine, braided, nonabsorbable material. The anastomosis is started by placing a single suture at two points which divide as accurately as possible the circumferences of graft and artery into two equal halves. Inasmuch as there will usually be some discrepancy in the circumference of the graft and the artery, this maneuver divides the responsibility for overcoming the discrepancy between the two halves of the suture line.

As the over-and-over anastomosis suture line is carried around the vessel (*C* and *D*), the individual sutures are placed about 2 mm. apart and about the same distance from the edge of the vessel. The discrepancy in circumference of the ends being connected is progressively reduced by each suture. The tension placed on the sutures is only that which brings the tissues together, and any degree of pursestringing of the suture line is avoided.

The posterior or far side of the distal suture line (*E* and *F*) may be placed from within without disadvantage, if rotation of the anastomosis line is difficult. Rotation makes the placement of this part of the distal suture simpler. The anastomosis is completed as shown in *G*.

Formation of thrombi distal to the point at which the repair is being done is minimized by the injection of a dilute heparin-saline solution. Any clots which may have formed either above or below the area must be removed before the final sutures are placed.

PLATE 14

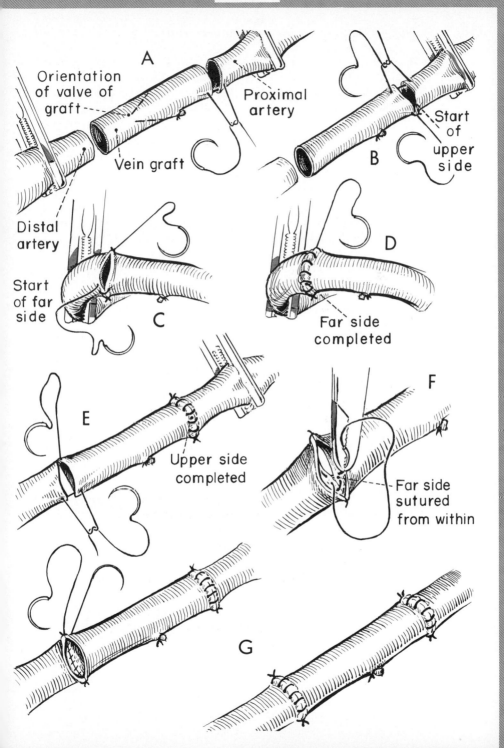

A

Orientation
of valve of
graft

Proximal
artery

Vein graft

Distal
artery

Start
of far
side

B

Start
of
upper
side

C

D

Far side
completed

E

Upper side
completed

F

Far side
sutured
from within

G

Wounds of an artery produced by a stab wound or by small projectiles ordinarily cause hemorrhage into the tissues rather than external bleeding. A pulsating hematoma or false aneurysm is produced when the hemorrhage is confined by tissue spaces and the hematoma remains in communication with the open arterial wound. A traumatic arteriovenous fistula is formed when the wound involves the artery and the adjacent vein. Both types of lesion are commonly encountered in the same injury.

The stab wound diagrammed in *A* shows penetration of the superficial femoral artery. *B* depicts the establishment of a false aneurysm or pulsating hematoma. The traumatic orifice of the artery communicates with a hematoma confined within the muscle and fascial layers of the thigh. Blood enters the hematoma during systole, due to the systolic blood pressure, and leaves the hematoma to re-enter the artery during diastole. The hematoma can be felt to pulsate, and the flow of blood through the orifice is audible with the stethoscope. The bruit may be heard only during systole or during both systole and diastole. If the latter is true, the bruit will not be continuous but, rather, will be interrupted at the end of systole and again at end of diastole when flow through the orifice is stopped as the direction of flow reverses.

In a traumatic arteriovenous fistula (*C*), the flow from artery to vein is continuous and always in one direction. It is more rapid during systole than during diastole, and the resulting bruit is continuous and has a characteristic machinery quality due to the systolic accentuation. The flow from artery to vein may not be established immediately after the injury but rather may become evident hours or days later. The common combination of pulsating hematoma and arteriovenous fistula is shown in *D*. In this lesion a pulsating mass is present, and in addition the characteristic continuous murmur of the fistula is audible.

PLATE 15

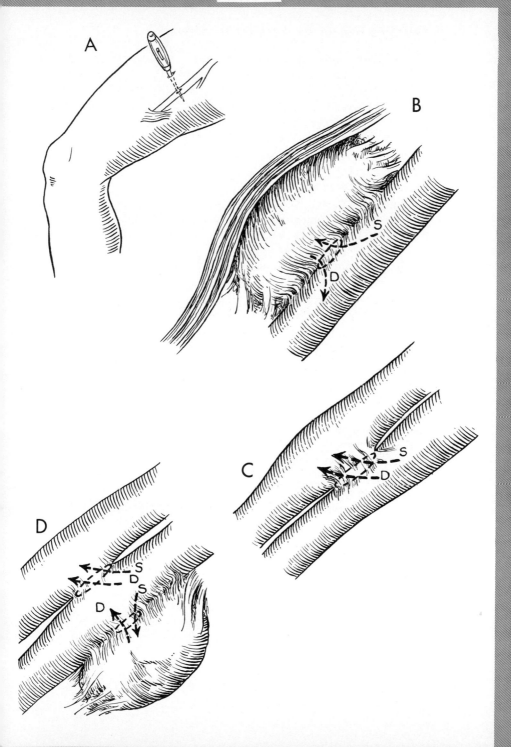

Immediate repair of arterial injuries is the accepted standard in surgery of trauma. Following this principle, the penetrating wound or small laceration of an artery that is likely to produce a pulsating hematoma would be repaired before this lesion was established in all of its characteristics. Immediate repair is indicated even if there is strong indication that a pulsating hematoma will form, despite the fact that this lesion can for a time be well tolerated. The false aneurysm may not follow a benign course; instead it may cause severe pain by compression of tissues, rupture to the outside through the external wound, or by its size and position obstruct the flow of blood through the artery of origin. If immediate repair is missed, delayed surgery should be avoided during the ensuing 12–14 days because of the possibility of infection and because there is during this time a distinct softening of a significant segment of the injured artery which makes sutures insecure.

A shows diagrammatically a pulsating hematoma in the popliteal area which has been present three years. It is characteristic of this lesion that it appears to involve a longer arterial segment than it actually does, because of adhesions between the hematoma and the external surface of the vessel. This relationship is shown in *B*, which also indicates the development of a smooth lining in the hematoma in continuity with the intima of the parent artery. After proximal and distal control of the artery has been obtained (*C*), dissection is carried out between the hematoma and the vessel in order to preserve arterial length. This maneuver is greatly aided by opening the hematoma. The arterial continuity may be re-established (*D*) by direct anastomosis, or sufficient artery may be lost to require a graft.

PLATE 16

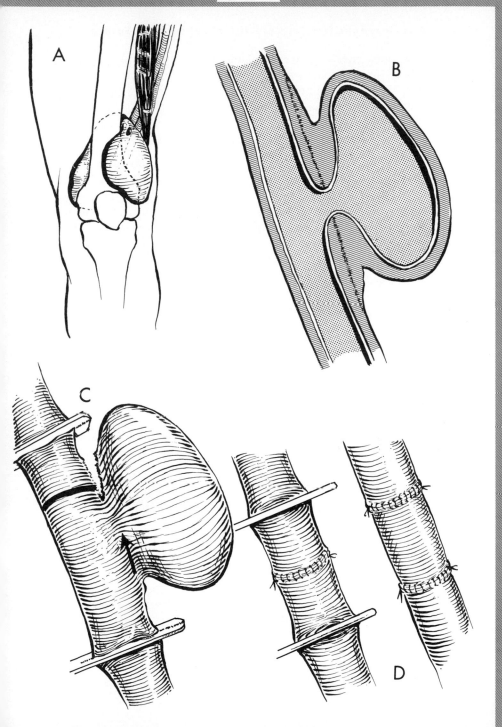

Various methods are available for the cure of arteriovenous fistula. These include resection after ligation of all of the arterial and venous components, repair of the ostium of the fistula, and resection with repair of the artery by anastomosis or graft.

Quadrilateral Ligation and Resection

An arteriovenous fistula stimulates the formation of both arterial and venous collaterals to a remarkable degree. Therefore, resection of the fistula is well tolerated so far as the preservation of tissues is concerned. However, if the fistula is in a major vessel, some degree of deficiency in arterial supply will almost certainly be manifest even though tissue is not lost. Quadrilateral ligation and excision should, therefore, be reserved for fistulas in relatively unimportant arteries.

In *A*, an arteriovenous fistula with pulsating hematoma is present as a compound lesion of the posterior tibial artery. The extent of the hematoma is indicated by the stippled area. The characteristic dilatation and tendency to elongation of the veins in communication with the fistula are shown. Proximal and then distal control of the artery above and below the fistula is followed by dissection of the venous side of the lesion with the arterial limbs either temporarily or finally occluded. The only serious difficulty in dissection usually encountered is in localizing and ligating the enlarged vein together with the branches of the vein in this area, all of which have acquired a significant size because of the high flow (*B*).

Transvenous Repair of Fistulous Opening

An arteriovenous fistula may be repaired by direct suture of the opening in the artery. The steps of proximal and distal control of both vessels in the region of the fistula are required. Scar tissue resulting from the original trauma is shown in *C* in a fistula between the superficial femoral artery and vein. The scar tissue is dissected with the least difficulty by following closely the arterial wall. After the vein and artery are completely isolated and provisionally occluded (*D*), the fistulous opening in the artery is visualized through an incision in the vein. Direct closure, as illustrated in *D* and *E*, can be done only if the fistulous opening is small.

PLATE 17

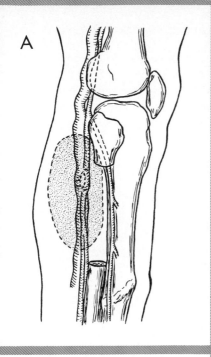

A

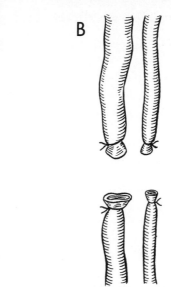

B

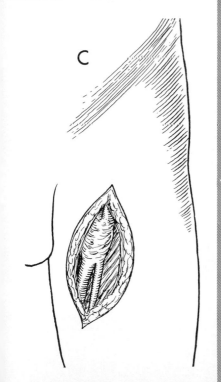

C

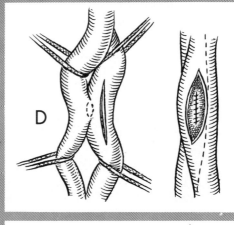

D

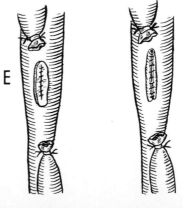

E

The standard repair of an arteriovenous fistula by end-to-end anastomosis of the artery after resection of the lesion takes advantage of the fact that very little of the artery, which is imbedded in scar tissue in the region of the injury, need be sacrificed if the fibrotic tissue surrounding it is dissected away. A fistula in which apparent damage to the artery extends for 2–3 in. is illustrated in *A*. The artery proximal and distal to the fistula has been controlled and is lifted by tapes. The pathologically enlarged vein is similarly exposed. After the artery has been freed to a point close to the fistula, it is occluded and the venous contributors to the lesion are carefully exposed and ligated (*B*).

Avoidance of troublesome bleeding during the repair depends upon identifying and ligating the surprisingly large number of veins of significant size. This is best done with the veins under only normal venous pressure after the arterial limbs have been obstructed. Repeated application and removal of the arterial clamps should be avoided because of the effect of the fistula on cardiac dynamics. Particularly to be avoided is occlusion of the distal artery while the proximal limb continues to function through the fistula because of the increase in cardiac venous return which will exist while such occlusion is present.

After occlusion of the four limbs of the fistula, dissection of the scar tissue is carried out very close to the arterial wall, where a plane of dissection seemingly in or beneath the adventitial layer exists. In *C* the provisional control of the vein is shown, and the permanent ligatures of the vein are in place but not tied as this dissection of the artery is carried out. A defect only 1–2 cm. in actual length (*D*) may be the result, and a direct end-to-end anastomosis can be done without undue tension (*E*). Secure ligation of the venous ends is essential, and simple ligation should be reinforced with a transfixing suture ligature.

PLATE 18

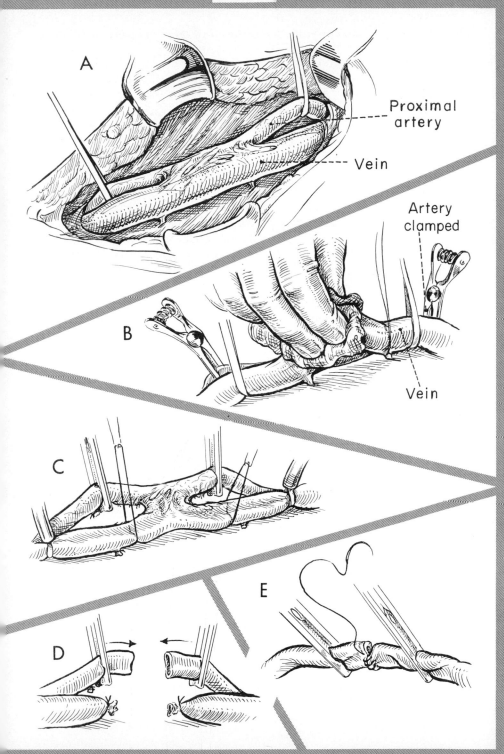

A

Proximal artery

Vein

Artery clamped

B

Vein

C

D

E

A variety of situations requires the use of a graft or prosthesis for restoration of arterial flow after removal of an arteriovenous fistula. These include the presence of unusually extensive original damage to the artery, damage to the artery during the difficult dissection, lack of elasticity of the artery due to the presence of arteriosclerosis, and aneurysm formation as a result of the increased blood flow stimulated by the fistula. The last indication is diagrammed in *A*.

In arteriovenous fistula it is typical that the proximal artery be enlarged. Occasionally this may be of aneurysmal proportion. If the stretching of the proximal artery has been unusually great, it may continue even after repair of the fistula because of fragmentation of the elastic layers of the vessel. Such a remarkable degree of enlargement of the vessel has been encountered principally in the iliac system proximal to a fistula in the region of Poupart's ligament, as illustrated here.

Application of the first principle in approaching an arterial lesion, namely, of proximal control, in this instance required isolation of the distal abdominal aorta and the opposite iliac artery. This is most easily carried out through a transabdominal incision. It can also be done without undue difficulty through an extraperitoneal approach using an oblique incision in the lower quadrant of the abdomen. Distal control through a longitudinal incision in the femoral triangle involved isolating the superficial femoral artery and the profunda femoris artery.

The entire dilated segment of the iliac and common femoral arteries was resected (*B*). The internal iliac artery is illustrated as being sacrificed, while the profunda femoris artery was anastomosed end-to-side to the graft as a final stage in the repair. The vein itself was securely ligated as close as possible to the fistula. Even though the vein is large and seems important, venous insufficiency need not be anticipated because of the characteristic massive development of venous channels in response to the fistula.

PLATE 19

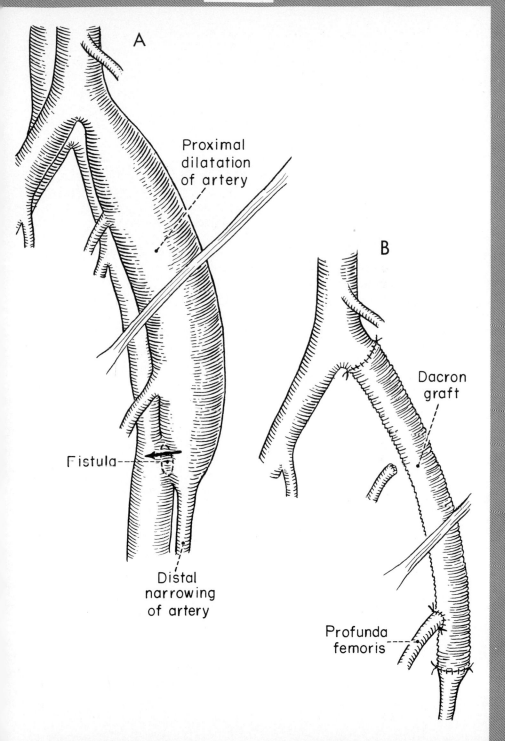

A

Proximal
dilatation
of artery

B

Fistula

Dacron
graft

Distal
narrowing
of artery

Profunda
femoris

CHAPTER 4

Acute Arterial Occlusion

AN ACUTE arterial occlusion other than that caused by trauma results either from an embolus or from the development in situ of a thrombus obstructing the lumen of the vessel. Thrombosis of a previously normal artery, though rare, is encountered in patients with polycythemia vera and polycythemia due to cyanotic congenital heart disease. Persons with polycythemia secondary to emphysema or other chronic pulmonary disease are predominantly in the arteriosclerotic age group and the arterial thrombosis probably would be in an area of previous disease.

Symptoms of an acute arterial occlusion consist of pain and loss of function. The pain is most often severe and continuous. The loss of function is both motor and sensory and develops soon after the acute occlusion occurs. Examination confirms the absence of sensory and motor function. The skin of the part is pale. The veins are collapsed and there is mild cyanosis, particularly marked in the nail beds. Several factors may be considered in evaluating the level at which pulsations are absent in terms of the level of the acute occlusion. Particularly in relation to embolism, these factors are: the great likelihood that the embolus is lodged in a major bifurcation; that lodgment of an embolus ordinarily produces a great deal of reflex arterial spasm, and, finally, that a quite strong pulse may be transmitted by the embolus itself and the position of the occlusion be misinterpreted as being at a lower level. In thrombosis of a previously diseased artery, the level of loss of pulse is more reliable as an indication of level of occlusion. Further, the occlusion is most apt to occur at those points in the arterial system in which arteriosclerotic changes predominate, namely, the major bifurcations and such areas of tendinous constriction as the upper adductor canal.

Differentiation between an embolic occlusion and a thrombosis of an arteriosclerotic segment is important because embolectomy is technically a less demanding procedure, so far as equipment and technical experience with vascular surgery are concerned, than are the procedures required to relieve an arteriosclerotic obstruction. Since surgical relief of the acute obstruction is indicated in either condition, differentiation has little bearing on the decision that surgery should or should not be done. The severity of the symptoms and signs of acute occlusion is greater in embolism because of the reflex constriction generated by the impact of the lodgment and because the occluded vessel is usually a normal one. The symptoms of thrombosis of a previously diseased artery depend on the amount of chronic obstruction that existed previously. If the lumen was severely stenosed before the final occluding thrombosis occurred and abundant collateral channels had developed, the acute episode may be unnoticed. The history of symptoms of chronic arterial insufficiency, such as intermittent claudication, and signs of chronic arterial disease in other regions aid in the differentiation. The presence of one of the cardiac lesions which most often are the sources of a peripheral arterial embolus is also of assistance in differential diagnosis. The presence of factors that favor both conditions need not be entirely misleading, because a patient with an area of arteriosclerosis in the lower extremity who has auricular fibrillation as the result of arteriosclerotic heart disease may very well have an embolus at the partially occluded point.

The aim of surgical therapy is the restoration of normal blood flow. The procedure to accomplish this is relatively simple in embolism and difficult in acute thrombotic occlusion. In the latter, simple removal of the thrombus is not sufficient, because the local condition would immediately cause a recurrence. Embolectomy is indicated in the case of embolic occlusion, but arterial reconstruction, not thrombectomy, is needed in most instances of thrombosis. The technique of embolectomy at various sites is described in the following plates. Arterial reconstruction is considered in Chapter 5, Chronic Arterial Occlusion.

Most peripheral arterial emboli result from the dislodgment of intracardiac thrombi. *A* shows the intracardiac lesions which are prone to produce clots. A left atrial thrombus may be suspected in the presence of atrial fibrillation with or without mitral valve disease or in the presence of mitral stenosis alone. Vegetations due to subacute bacterial endocarditis of the mitral or aortic valves usually produce small emboli which carry with them the etiologic bacteria of the initial lesion and, therefore, cause not only obstruction in smaller vessels, but infection at the site of lodgment. Tumors (myxoma) of the left atrium may also be a source of emboli. The internal surface of a myocardial infarct often develops a covering of mural thrombus which, if it gives rise to embolism, characteristically dislodges some days following the acute myocardial episode.

Also shown in *A* is the route taken by a blood clot arising in a peripheral vein. After entering the right atrium, the clot may go through an interatrial septal defect or a patent foramen ovale to become a systemic rather than a pulmonary arterial embolus.

Atheromatous debris at the carotid bifurcation may embolize to the brain (*B*). Popliteal aneurysms may be a common source of emboli to the distal leg and foot (*C*). The mural thrombus within an aneurysm of the abdominal aorta or a portion of atheromatous plaque or a thrombus developing in an ulceration of the abdominal aorta in atherosclerosis (*D*) occasionally acts as the source of emboli to the lower extremities.

PLATE 20

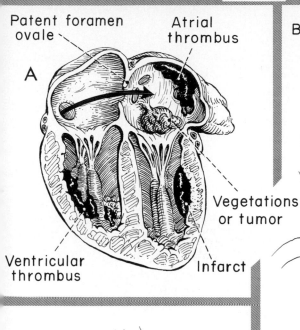

A

Patent foramen ovale

Atrial thrombus

Vegetations or tumor

Ventricular thrombus

Infarct

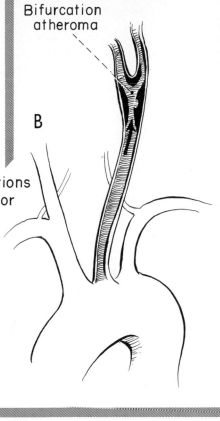

B

Bifurcation atheroma

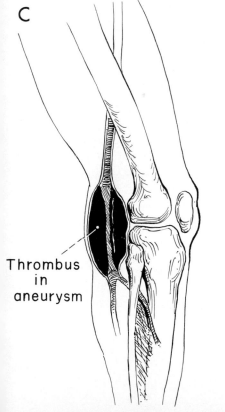

C

Thrombus in aneurysm

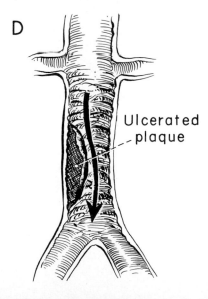

D

Ulcerated plaque

Removal of the occluding embolus with restoration of normal blood flow should be the object of treatment in every instance except that of involvement of very small vessels in which the principal cause of symptoms is reflex arterial spasm. The embolectomy should be done at the earliest possible time, but a distinct time limit as such cannot be set. The development of ischemic tissue changes, through which re-establishment of circulation might be dangerous, is the rather indefinite limiting factor. Peripheral emboli can almost without exception be removed using local anesthesia. Removal can be carried out, therefore, on all except the most seriously ill cardiac patients. Removal of emboli of the abdominal visceral arteries or of the aortic bifurcation, although more strenuous for the patient, is most strongly indicated because such obstructions are usually fatal if untreated.

Reflex arterial spasm is responsible for much of the pain in embolism and for some of the ischemia. Formerly, much emphasis was placed on doing a sympathetic nerve block prior to arterial embolectomy. In recent years this is rarely, if ever, done. Anticoagulation in the form of heparinization is considered extremely important before surgery. Immediate surgery is the treatment of choice.

INCISIONS FOR EMBOLECTOMY

Locations of the incisions through which emboli are commonly removed are indicated in Plate 21. These locations reflect the fact that most emboli lodge at major branches or bifurcations of the arteries involved.

It is important to be prepared to explore the bifurcations distal to the one at which the embolus is primarily lodged because of the tendency of an embolus to break up and a fragment to pass on to the next branch of the artery. For example, the entire lower extremity must be prepared and draped when removing a femoral bifurcation embolus, so that pieces at the popliteal bifurcation can be removed directly and thrombi within the branches of the popliteal artery can be flushed out through incisions in the arteries at the ankle level if necessary. The same considerations dictate preparation of the entire upper extremity when embolectomy is done at the innominate, subclavian or brachial level.

PLATE 21

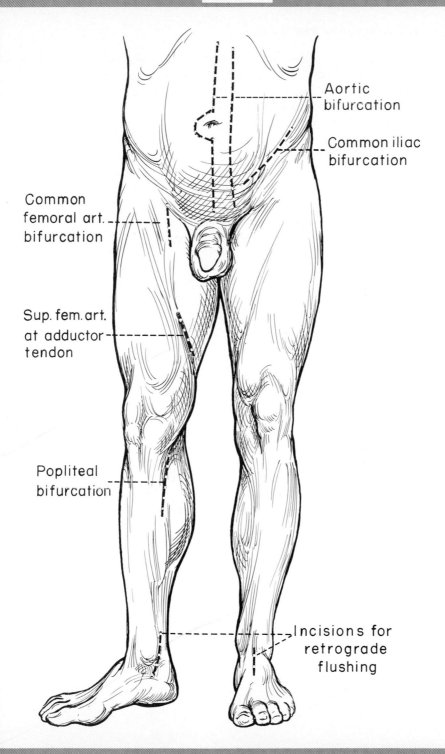

Aortic
bifurcation

Common iliac
bifurcation

Common
femoral art.
bifurcation

Sup. fem. art.
at adductor
tendon

Popliteal
bifurcation

Incisions for
retrograde
flushing

The primary step in any embolectomy consists in preparation of the part involved so that any accessible portion of the arterial system beyond the point of primary occlusion can be approached without redraping. The second step consists in obtaining control of the obstructed artery and its branches above and below the point of embolic occlusion. The introduction of the balloon catheter as advocated by Fogarty to remove a propagating thrombus has revolutionized the surgical approach to embolectomy. If the balloon catheter is not available, the clot is removed through an arteriotomy wound and the distal propagating thrombus may be removed by suction or by distal flushing in a retrograde fashion.

A shows the exposure of the common femoral bifurcation through a longitudinal incision in the femoral triangle. Also shown is the anterior medial approach to the popliteal bifurcation with the balloon catheter. Often only one incision is needed, that for the exposure of the common femoral. The balloon catheter may be passed all the way to the foot in this manner and any propagating thrombus removed. Occasionally, however, the popliteal artery will need to be exposed.

B is a close-up view of the common femoral bifurcation, showing the arteriotomy incision made directly over the embolus itself. *C* illustrates the removal with forceps of the embolus with thrombus casts from the profunda and superficial femoral arteries. In *D* the extraction of the distal propagating thrombus by the balloon catheter through the common femoral arteriotomy is seen.

Following removal of the embolus and the propagating thrombus, heparin solution may be instilled distally, although all these patients are heparinized systemically prior to surgery. The arteriotomies are closed in the usual fashion with continuous 5 – 0 silk or Dacron-Teflon suture material.

Transverse arteriotomy is preferred in many instances to the longitudinal incision shown in this illustration. The size and character of the artery may influence one's decision as to what type of incision to use.

PLATE 22

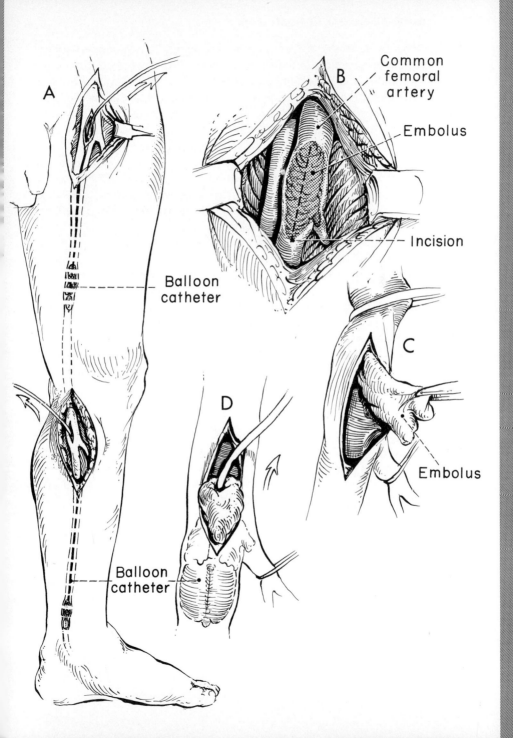

A

B — Common femoral artery

Embolus

Incision

C

Embolus

D

Balloon catheter

Balloon catheter

The skin of the lower extremities should be given complete surgical preparation in addition to preparation of the abdomen, so that the distal vessels can be exposed if necessary. With the advent of the balloon catheter, in almost every instance aortic bifurcation embolectomy is possible from below through incisions in the common femoral arteries exposed under local anesthesia. Unless a portion of the embolus has broken loose at the time of impact above, the vessels will be found to be soft and pulseless. Each common femoral artery is freed from its bed and elevated with tapes (*A*). An arteriotomy incision is made in each common femoral artery large enough to admit the catheter and to release the inflated balloon when it is pulled out of the artery.

The balloon catheter is passed up one limb to a point above the bifurcation of the aorta (*B*). While this is being done, a bulldog clamp may be placed on the other common femoral artery to prevent any distal passage of clots that may be dislodged by this maneuver. The balloon is inflated, and the catheter is then pulled distally, extracting the clots through the incision in the common femoral artery (*C*). A similar procedure is repeated on the contralateral side, removing all clots possible (*D*). It is often necessary to repeat the procedure several times to remove the embolus and propagating thrombus thoroughly. Even the advent of vigorous bleeding may not indicate complete removal of clots.

Following good pulse flow to the groin bilaterally, clamps are placed on the common femoral artery. The balloon catheter, which is usually of a smaller size for use distally, is then passed through the superficial femoral artery as well as past the popliteal bifurcation into the lower leg. Gentle traction is applied after careful inflation of the balloon. The resistance to the passage of the balloon is carefully sensed by the operator's fingers as he withdraws the balloon catheter. Again, several passages may be necessary to ensure complete removal of the distal propagating thrombus. Following re-establishment of flow, good pulses should be felt at the ankle; if they are not, strong consideration should be given to exposure of the popliteal artery to make sure that there is no remaining clot at this point.

PLATE 23

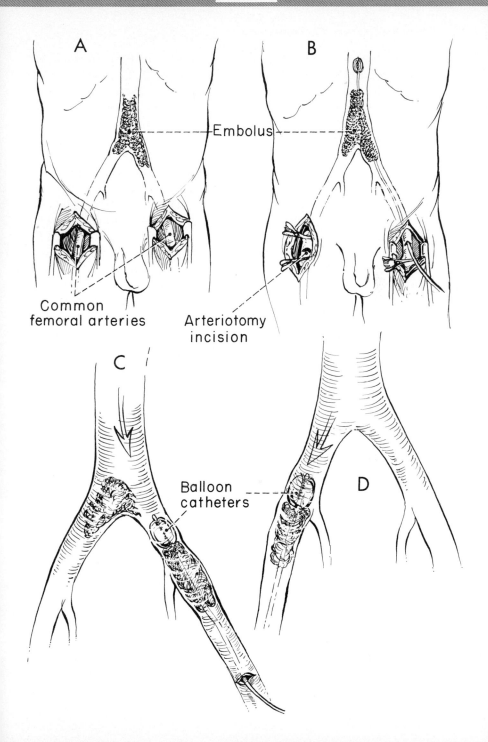

A

B

Embolus

Common
femoral arteries

Arteriotomy
incision

C

Balloon
catheters

D

Embolism of the brachial artery occurs more frequently at the origin of the deep brachial artery than it does at the bifurcation of the brachial artery at the elbow. The exposure of the vessel under local anesthesia is not difficult in either location. Its exposure at the more common site of occlusion is shown in *A*.

The longitudinal incision is made in the sulcus between the triceps and biceps muscle groups, centering on the point of termination of the palpable pulse. This point is usually easily found by palpation. In this area the artery lies beneath the brachial vein and is closely related to the median nerve which lies anterior and the ulnar nerve which lies posterior to it (*A*); these structures are separated from the artery. Proximal and distal control is obtained and a longitudinal incision is made in the brachial artery over the embolus (*B*).

A balloon catheter is passed proximally into the brachioaxillary artery (*C*), and the embolus and proximal thrombus are removed with the inflated balloon. The balloon catheter is then passed distally (*D*) and the distal propagating thrombus is removed. The distal artery is flushed with heparin solution, and the arteriotomy is closed in the usual manner with 5 – 0 silk or Teflon-Dacron suture material.

Before terminating the procedure, the operator must make sure a distal pulse is felt. If it is not, more distal exposure of the artery is indicated.

PLATE 24

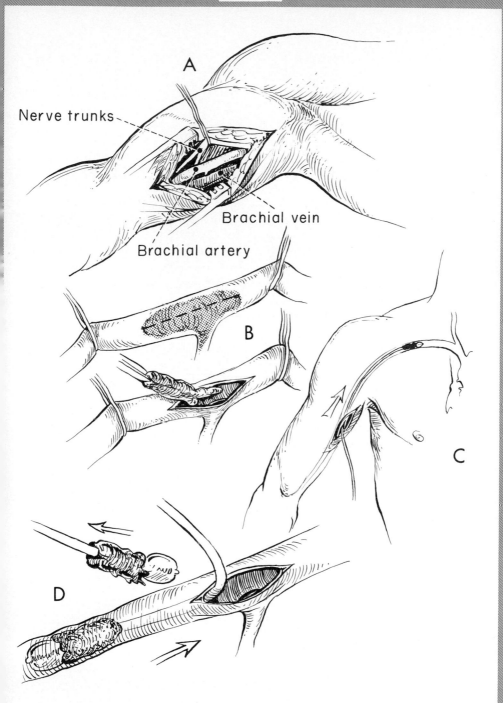

Nerve trunks

Brachial vein

Brachial artery

A

B

C

D

CHAPTER 5

Chronic Arterial Occlusion

THE COMMON ETIOLOGY of slowly developing arterial occlusions is the group of lesions classed together as arteriosclerosis. Results of reconstructive arterial surgery have been favorable in varying degrees in most regions in which large arteries become obstructed in a segmental fashion. Success has been greatest in the vessels of largest caliber, such as the aorta. Smaller vessels of major importance—for example, the renal arteries—can be successfully restored to function when the occluding lesion is contained within a short segment. Reconstructive surgery becomes more difficult and less likely to produce long-lasting benefit in more diffuse disease of medium-sized vessels, such as the femoral artery. Surgical restoration of the smaller vessels beyond the knee and elbow continues to offer a difficult problem.

In arterial insufficiency produced by a developing segmental occlusion, symptoms of a functional character usually appear long before tissue changes such as atrophy or loss of viability. The slower the process, the more truly this applies, because of the opportunity for maximum development of collateral channels. Thus, the patient with a segmental occlusion affecting the lower extremities will experience the functional symptom of intermittent claudication before there is atrophy or gangrene. The patient with renal artery stenosis shows the disturbance of function manifested by hypertension before there is irreversible damage to the kidney, and the patient with segmental stenosis of the extracranial cerebral arterial channels evidences symptoms and signs of intermittent cerebral ischemia before a brain infarct occurs.

Recognition of the meaning of claudication in the extremities, of such signs of intermittent cerebral ischemia as dizziness, transient blindness and transient muscular weakness, and of the special meaning of hypertension in some patients becomes important because of the surgical relief available for many of these potentially dangerous lesions.

Proper evaluation of physical signs and, in many cases, arterial visualization by x-ray serve as a basis for selection of patients for direct arterial surgery. Caution and conservatism are important in such selection, because the immediate failure of a reconstructive procedure may have disastrous results. Also, particularly in surgery of the femoral-popliteal area, late failure of an initially successful reconstruction is a serious matter because, during the period of restored circulation, atrophy occurs in the previously better developed collateral arterial bed.

The classic example of a slowly developing, complete occlusion of a segment of a major artery is that of the aortic bifurcation. During the gradual development of the obstruction, the enlargement of collateral arterial channels maintains flow at a level adequate for all nutritive requirements. However, the collaterals lack the ability to expand in response to the need for increased blood supply during exercise. The typical combination of intermittent claudication and normal nutrition results. The femoral pulses are initially palpable though diminished and possibly unequal. A bruit is audible over them. When the occlusion becomes complete the bruit disappears and a femoral pulse, if felt, is delayed and weak because it is transmitted by collateral channels.

Two general types of reconstructive procedures are used for segmental occlusion such as that at the aortic bifurcation. In one, the diseased inner portions of the arterial media and the thickened intima are removed from the vessel by careful dissection, leaving sufficient vessel wall for continued function without serious danger of dilatation. In the second, vascular grafts or substitutes are employed to re-establish normal arterial flow. Choice between thromboendarterectomy and graft is not based on inflexible indications.

In preparation for any reconstruction of the occluded aortic bifurcation, the lower extremities as well as the abdomen are prepared and draped. The aorta is exposed through a midline or right rectus abdominal incision. With the transverse mesocolon retracted upward and all loops of small bowel retracted to the right, often up out of the incision, the posterior parietal peritoneum is incised between the base of the small bowel mesentery on the right and the inferior mesenteric vein on the left, from the ligament of Treitz downward over the brim of the pelvis. The aorta is then exposed through this rather avascular area by sharp dissection, protecting the left renal vein which lies in these tissues at the upper end of the exposure (*A*). All branches arising from the segment of the vessels to be operated upon must be accurately located and controlled, either by small bulldog clamps or by doubly passed loops of medium-sized silk ligature material. A diagrammatic representation of the lesion is shown in *B*.

The aorta is shown cross-clamped at a level below the renal arteries in *C*. The aorta and the left common iliac artery are incised longitudinally in a continuous fashion, while a second, shorter arteriotomy is made in the right common iliac artery. Variations of this technique are used, including substitution of several transverse arteriotomy wounds for the longitudinal one. A plane of dissection is found in which the greatest possible amount of uninvolved media will be left to support the cleared channel. This dissection is carried out until the atheromatous material can all be removed.

If the edge left at the distal extremity of the thromboendarterectomy is prominent, it is carefully secured to the wall by interrupted fine sutures tied on the exterior of the vessel (*D*). *E* shows the repair of the arteriotomy wounds.

PLATE 25

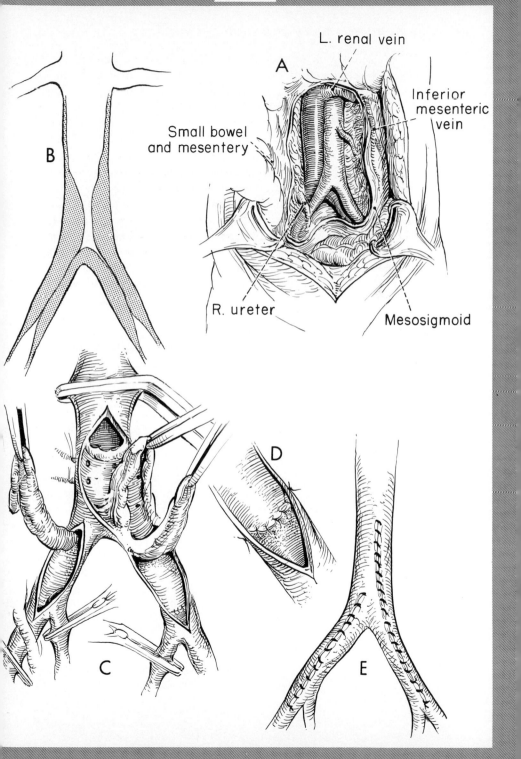

A

L. renal vein

Inferior mesenteric vein

Small bowel and mesentery

R. ureter

Mesosigmoid

B

C

D

E

The earliest use of a graft in treatment of occlusions of the aortic bifurcation consisted of actual substitution after complete removal of the diseased aortic bifurcation. Homologous aortic bifurcation grafts were standard replacements. Their use has now almost entirely been supplanted by synthetic grafts constructed of woven materials. These prostheses are directly loomed as bifurcations, and the Dacron or other artificial fibers of which they are made enable them to hold a circular crimping, which increases their flexibility. They are usually placed as by-passes, anastomosed end-to-side to the vessels above and below the occlusion.

The by-pass technique, illustrated in Plate 26, is applicable to any complete or partial occlusion of the aortic bifurcation. It is particularly desirable when the obstruction is incomplete, as in the example shown in *A*. Flow through the remaining lumen of the diseased segment is interrupted for only brief periods or perhaps not at all. This technique of by-pass of the abdominal aorta is used less frequently in present-day management. It should be used with very localized lesions at the bifurcation when endarterectomy is not decided upon, and particularly if the proximal aorta distal to the renal arteries is of excellent quality.

The aorta is exposed up to the level of the left renal vein, which is seen coursing across the aorta to enter the vena cava in *B*. A curved clamp is then applied for partial exclusion of a generous portion of the anterior wall of the aorta to permit a longitudinal incision to be made for the end-to-side anastomosis of the upper end of the bifurcation graft. This procedure takes advantage of the usual relative lack of involvement of the anterior surface of the vessel. If it appears hazardous to apply this clamp, a segment of the aorta at this level of sufficient length for arteriotomy and anastomosis to the graft may be isolated between transversely placed clamps. The end of the prosthesis, which is beveled, is sutured to the longitudinal arteriotomy with an over-and-over suture of Teflon-Dacron. This anastomosis is started at the upper and lower ends (*C* and *D*), one suture being used for each side. The suture line on one side of the aortotomy incision has been completed in *E*.

[Aortic bifurcation by-pass *continued on page 86.*]

PLATE 26

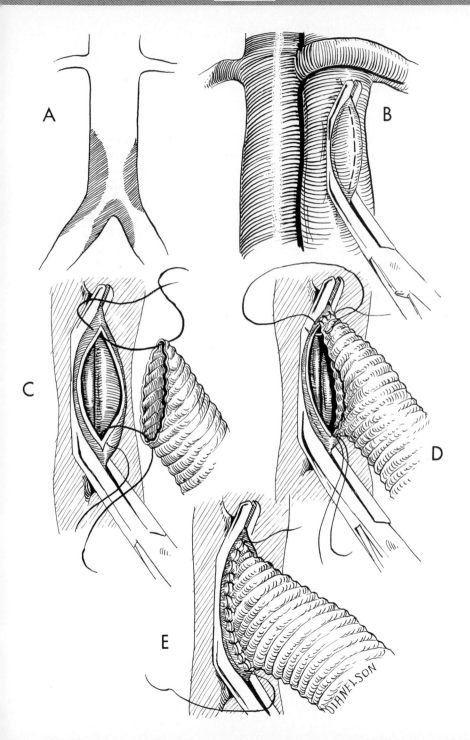

In *F*, the second suture line of the proximal anastomosis to the aorta is being started. After the proximal anastomosis is completed (*G*), the distal sites of the anastomosis are selected and both iliac limbs of the bifurcation prosthesis are trimmed to proper length. The same type of anastomosis is used for the distal end-to-side anastomoses into the external iliac arteries (*H*). Heparin is usually administered systemically just prior to the clamping of the aorta.

In *I*, all anastomoses have been completed and the clamps removed, with circulation restored by way of the prosthesis.

Most crimped, woven prostheses commonly available are of sufficient porosity to require preclotting with blood drawn from the patient before implantation is begun. Also, it is important to draw this blood prior to heparinization. Occasionally, even with supposedly adequate preclotting, there may be instances of bleeding through the graft itself. This is either due to a defect in the graft or to some unusual reaction to heparin. The heparin may be neutralized with protamine. If bleeding still persists, unusual measures, such as wrapping the graft with another piece of Dacron cloth, may be necessary to stop the bleeding.

[Aortic bifurcation by-pass with end-to-end proximal anastomosis *on page 88.*]

PLATE 26

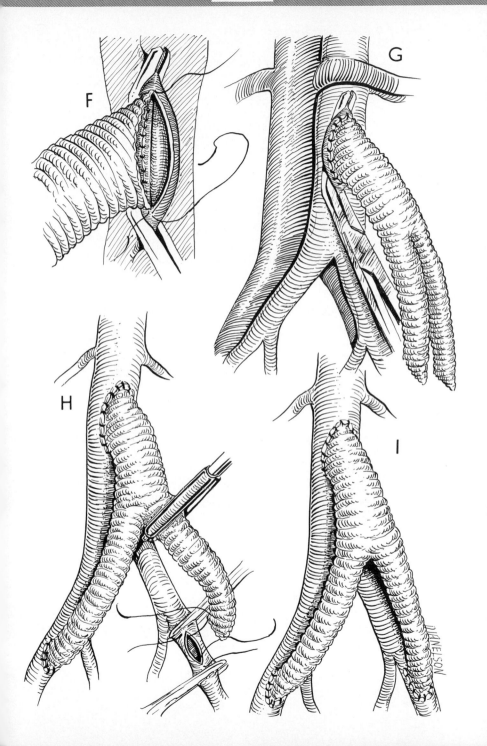

End-to-End Proximal Anastomosis

The use of a prosthetic device to by-pass the obstructed aortic bifurcation allows for variation both at the proximal site of anastomosis and at the distal sites.

A shows the completed exposure of the abdominal aorta and its bifurcation. The left renal vein is shown coursing in front of the aorta and entering the vena cava, which is only partly exposed to the right of the aorta. The left renal artery is seen in its usual position in relation to the renal vein. In this instance, the thrombus within the aorta proximal to the complete occlusion at the bifurcation extended up to the level of the renal arteries. Clot in this region, or even atheromas about the orifices of the renal arteries, can be removed through the cut end of the aorta, transected below the renal orifices.

In *B* the aorta is shown occluded with an arterial clamp above the origin of the renal arteries. The left renal vein is elevated sharply to gain exposure. Care is required to avoid long obstruction of this vein unless the renal artery is also obstructed. The aorta has been transected, and clot is being taken from the posterior aortic wall and from the left renal artery. When both renal arteries have been cleared and it has been amply demonstrated that there is no clot above the aortic clamp, the aortic occlusion is moved down to a point below the renal artery origins (*C*) and the proximal end-to-end anastomosis is done.

The duration of renal ischemia should be minimized and, unless unusual difficulty is encountered in clearing the renal segment of the aorta, will not be in excess of 15 minutes. Injection of dilute heparin solution into the aorta just as the clamp is being placed in its first position may be desirable to discourage thrombosis of small renal artery branches.

The proximal end of the distal portion of the aorta is very securely closed with two layers of suture (*B*) after renal artery flow has been re-established. This should be done before the distal anastomoses hold the graft down in the field.

In the method of anastomosis shown in *C*, both sutures are started posteriorly and carried around to be completed anteriorly. This minimizes manipulation of the aorta end which is often fragile.

[Aortic bifurcation by-pass *continued on page 90.*]

PLATE 27

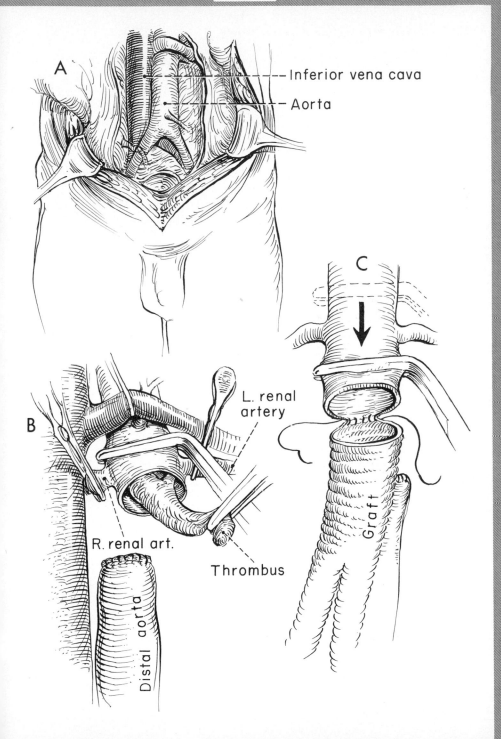

A

—————— Inferior vena cava

—————— Aorta

C

B

L. renal artery

R. renal art.

Thrombus

Distal aorta

Graft

Selection of a site suitable for the implantation of the distal limbs of the bifurcation prosthesis depends on the presence of vessel walls suitable for anastomosis and on the certainty that the occluding lesion will be completely by-passed. At times the anastomosis can be made at the distal common iliac. This is more often true in aneurysms than it is in occlusive disease, however. Many times anastomosis is made end-to-side to the external iliac artery and if necessary, of course, is carried down to the common femoral below. Contrary to early experience, grafts are not carried beyond the common femoral level as one continuous graft. They are, however, very satisfactory to the common femoral level, anastomosed either to the common femoral itself or to the combination of the common femoral and profunda femoris.

D shows the graft being trimmed to the proper size after the level of anastomosis has been decided. In *E* and *F*, the anastomosis is carried out on one side of the distal common iliac artery. The graft is then allowed to fill with blood from below through the completed anastomosis (*G*). Blood flow is established into the completed side after evacuation of any possible clots from the aorta above (*H*).

PLATE 27

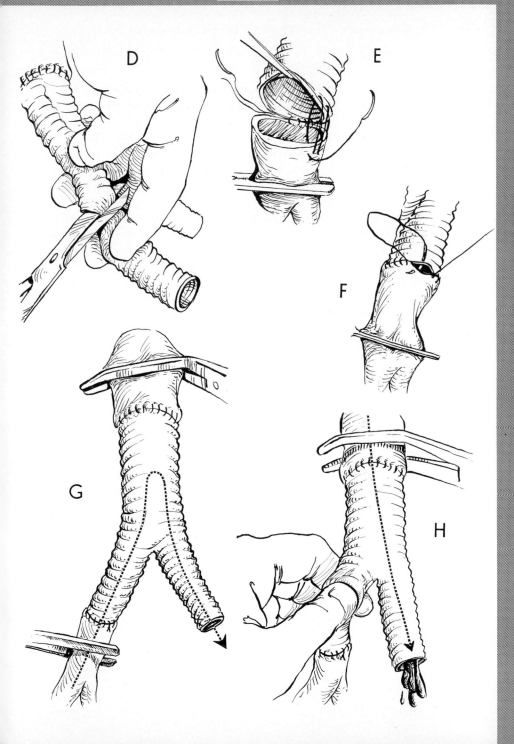

PROFUNDA REVASCULARIZATION

If a patient has both aortoiliac disease and superficial femoral blocks, it is best to do the revascularization to the profunda level as a first-stage procedure. In many instances this is all that is necessary to restore a good collateral pulse at the ankle. The concept of "profunda revascularization" is a very important one. When extensive aortoiliac disease is present, one may accomplish revascularization either by an extensive endarterectomy or with a by-pass graft such as that illustrated in Plate 28.

Both common femoral arteries and their bifurcations are exposed (*A*) and rather extensive dissection of the profunda femoris artery undertaken. The aorta has been exposed above and the most common type of anastomosis, that is, an end-to-end to the aorta above with oversewing of the distal aorta, is carried out.

Tunneling is accomplished under the inguinal ligament and the graft is brought down into the common femoral area (*B*). The anastomosis may be made directly to the common femoral artery if it is minimally diseased. If there is extensive disease in the common femoral artery as well as major involvement of the profunda femoris, an endarterectomy of the common femoral and the profunda femoris artery is performed (*C*). It is important to dissect the branches of the profunda femoris so that endarterectomy of the artery terminates in a normal artery. When a long incision extending from the common femoral into the profunda has been made, the end of the graft may be cut to form an elongated patch to widen the entire lumen (*D*).

AXILLOFEMORAL BY-PASS.—In very poor-risk patients one may choose not to do an extensive bifurcation graft but to bring a graft from the axillary artery subcutaneously down to the femoral level and/or to the profunda femoris. This operation may be done under light general anesthesia and avoids abdominal exploration. Variations of the axillofemoral by-pass may be a graft from the one axillofemoral graft to the opposite femoral artery. This procedure is also useful in problems of infected grafts when a by-pass of the infected area is necessary. In addition, grafts may be brought from the opposite femoral artery—if the pulsation is good in the opposite side—to revascularize the extremity with an occluded iliac.

PLATE 28

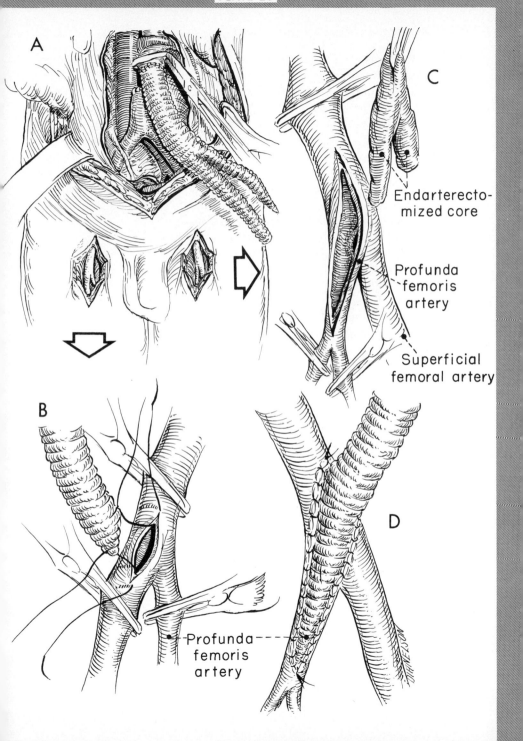

A

B

C

Endarterecto-
mized core

Profunda
femoris
artery

Superficial
femoral artery

D

Profunda
femoris
artery

Whenever possible, the choice of graft in a femoropopliteal by-pass reconstruction is an autogenous saphenous vein graft. The only limitation in the choice of this graft is its size and, therefore, on occasions it may not be possible to use it. The saphenous vein is usually obtained from the same leg through several incisions, including the operative incision, with ligation of its branches and distention of the vein graft by pressure. The vein graft is carefully trimmed of all loose adventitia and the ends fashioned for anastomosis. It is reversed to allow proper flow through the valves. In situ nonreversed grafts have been used, but not in our experience. In this case the valves must be destroyed.

If a vein graft is not suitable, an 8 – 10 mm. woven Dacron prosthesis may be used (Plate 30). Careful selection of cases is important when Dacron prostheses are used and it is preferable not to go beyond the knee joint unless it is absolutely necessary. Short grafts, of both the autogenous vein and Dacron types, are preferable to long grafts. Because of this, proximal endarterectomies of the superficial femoral may be done to reduce the length of graft.

A shows the proximal and distal exposure of the femoral upper popliteal artery in the typical adductor canal block. In *B*, the vein graft has been prepared; an incision is made in each end for the proper fastening of the graft for an end-to-side anastomosis. One technique of end-to-side anastomosis is shown in *C*, using a single suture at each end of the arteriotomy and a continuous suture along each side. *D* shows the completed by-pass vein graft.

PLATE 29

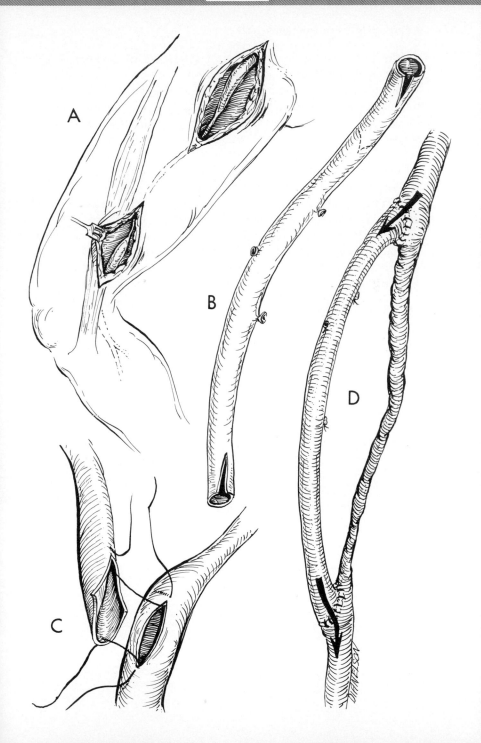

We have experienced a higher failure rate of crimped Dacron tube prostheses than of autogenous saphenous vein grafts placed as long by-passes or replacements in femoral artery reconstruction. The prosthesis has advantages, however, of being always available in any needed length and of requiring no additional dissection, as does a vein graft. It seems very important to be highly critical in selection of patients for femoral artery reconstruction so that, unless the segment of occlusion is quite short, only those with really significant symptoms be operated upon.

When a Dacron prosthesis is necessary, the optimum tube diameter is 8 mm. It is carefully preclotted, as previously described (p. 86). The exposure of the proximal and distal areas of the artery is that shown in *A*. In *B* and *C* a type of end-to-side anastomosis is shown that is begun with two sutures at one end and uses a continuous suture up both sides of the arteriotomy. *D* and *E* show the completed by-pass graft.

PLATE 30

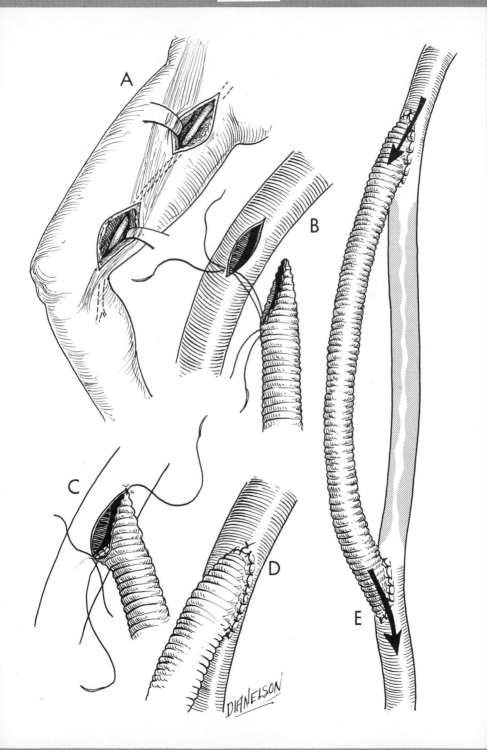

A

B

C

D

E

DIANELSON

The smaller diameter of the superficial femoral artery is a serious handicap to the application of open thromboendarterectomy such as that described for the aortic bifurcation (p. 82). This is in large measure due to the further reduction in vessel diameter produced by the suture closing the longitudinal arteriotomy. Implantation of a segment of the patient's saphenous vein, opened up and placed with intima inward, widens the repaired area. Seldom is the saphenous vein too small for use in this manner. The technique is illustrated at a very common occlusion site, the upper end of the adductor (Hunter's) canal.

The occluded segment is exposed through an incision directly over the adductor canal. The occluded segment is isolated and clamps are applied proximally and distally (*A*). The collaterals are encircled with heavy silk for temporary control. The endarterectomy is initiated as in *B* and is shown being completed in *C*. In *D* a close-up is shown of an intimal edge secured by interrupted sutures as it must be if it has significant thickness or shows a tendency to separate beyond the intended end of the endarterectomy. It is more desirable to have an endarterectomy completed in such a way that the end of the core is peeled smoothly from the artery. An autogenous vein patch graft is fashioned to fit the defect (*E*) and is sutured to the arteriotomy incision. Two sutures are placed at the end and a continuous suture is placed on each side of the arteriotomy until the patch is completely in place (*F* and *G*).

The technique may be applied to longer segments of occlusion. It is important not to make the patch too large, for there will be turbulence in the artificially dilated segment that results.

PLATE 31

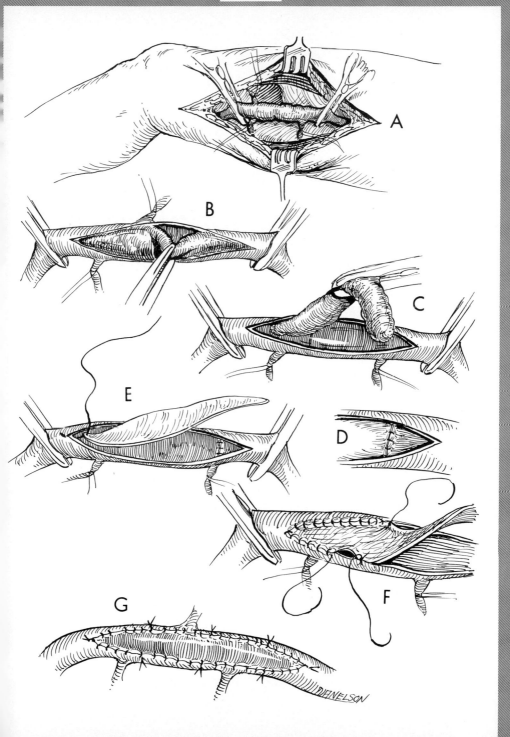

A

B

C

E

D

F

G

DIENELSON

CHAPTER 6

Surgical Aspects
of Coronary Artery Disease

SURGICAL CONTRIBUTIONS to the management of coronary arteriosclerosis now include direct and indirect techniques designed to increase myocardial blood supply and reconstructive procedures to correct certain complications of myocardial infarcts. There is, in addition, great promise in the development of surgical relief of acute coronary artery occlusions, thereby preventing an infarct, and of resectional therapy of infarcts during their early stages.

The development of surgical procedures for myocardial revascularization has been difficult and laborious. This has been due to lack of objective methods for evaluating the extent of arterial disease and the postoperative results. In the past few years, however, selective coronary angiography has afforded accurate estimation of coronary artery involvement, allowing the proper choice of surgical procedures. Postoperative evaluation by visualization of the internal mammary artery has confirmed beyond doubt the value of internal mammary implantation in demonstrating the abundant communications between the implant and the coronary artery system in some individuals. Coronary angiography has also demonstrated that the majority of patients with disabling ischemic heart disease have extensive involvement of the vessels, precluding the feasibility of direct reconstructive procedures.

The ideal candidate for myocardial revascularization by an implant is a relatively young individual with disabling angina at rest or on mild exertion in whom selective coronary angiography has demonstrated severe and diffuse occlusive disease. The presence of massive scar tissue in the myocardium due to repeated myocardial infarcts diminishes the likelihood of collateral formation. The choice between a single or a double internal mammary implant depends on the extent of arterial disease and myocardial ischemia.

Direct arterial surgery should be reserved for segmental lesions in the proximal portion of the major branches with arteries of adequate size beyond the obstruction. The use of a by-pass vein graft from the ascending aorta to the coronary artery distal to the atheromatous lesion is preferable to coronary artery endarterectomy and onlay patch graft, but both are in use.

Myocardial revascularization occasionally is indicated in combination with resection of ventricular aneurysm or valve replacement.

Although it is difficult to predict the value of coronary artery surgery in prolongation of life at this stage of development, there is no doubt that a satisfactory Vineberg implant or the restoration of coronary flow by a by-pass graft relieves the angina and improves the cardiac function.

The complications of infarct which are amenable to surgical treatment are ventricular aneurysm, rupture of a necrotic mitral papillary muscle with resulting detachment of one or several chordae tendineae and perforation of the ventricular septum through an infarct involving it.

The illustrations in this chapter will deal with the revascularization procedures and the technique of left ventricular aneurysm resection.

Revascularization of the anterior wall of the left ventricle is indicated in patients who have severe disabling angina pectoris and in whom selective coronary angiography has demonstrated an occlusive lesion of the anterior descending branch of the left coronary artery. The presence of massive scarring of the ventricle due to repeated myocardial infarction or the aneurysmal dilatation of the anterior wall of the left ventricle would make the possibility of collateral development less likely. Patients with diffuse arteriosclerotic changes of both right and left coronary arterial systems deserve bilateral implants to provide a new source for both anterior and posterior walls of the heart.

A single implant can be accomplished through a left thoracotomy. The patient is placed on the operating table in a lateral position, having the left side elevated about 45 degrees. Through a left anterolateral fifth intercostal space thoracotomy incision, the chest cavity is entered. The lung is retracted posteriorly, the internal mammary artery may be dissected entirely free from the sixth interspace upward (*A*) or be freed with surrounding tissues above the fourth rib (*C*). Careful dissection is required for proper control of bleeding from the intercostal branches of the internal mammary artery. After adequate dissection, the distal end of the internal mammary is transected (*A*), leaving several branches attached to the internal mammary in order to provide more bleeding points into the myocardial tunnel.

The pericardium is then incised anteriorly to the apex of the heart and the ischemic area of the ventricle is selected for the implantation of the internal mammary artery. With the use of a vascular clamp, a tunnel is constructed in the substance of the anterior wall of the left ventricle, taking the direction of the anterior descending branch (*B*). The internal mammary artery is implanted in the tunnel, particular care being taken to avoid constriction of the artery. Also, particular attention is required to avoid twisting of the internal mammary as it traverses the chest cage and enters the myocardium.

C and *D* show the same procedure, using the internal mammary with the Sewell modification. The pedicle can be sutured to the epicardium to secure it in place and to prevent twisting of the vessel.

PLATE 32

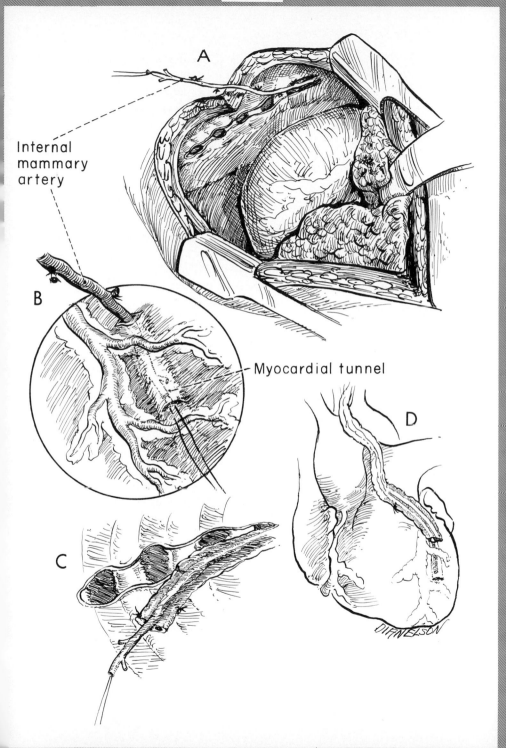

A

Internal
mammary
artery

B

Myocardial tunnel

C

D

DIFINELSON

Restoration of coronary flow by endarterectomy and onlay patch graft (Plate 34) should be reserved for patients who have a stenotic lesion with a relatively intact proximal end in a surgically accessible portion of the right or main left coronary artery. In patients with compromised flow in the proximal portion of the coronary artery and satisfactory lumen beyond the area of obstruction, an aorto-coronary by-pass is the procedure of choice.

A median sternotomy incision provides excellent exposure for an aorto-right coronary by-pass and is also used in patients whose lesion permits a distal anastomosis to the anterior descending branch. The left main coronary artery, however, is best exposed through a left anterolateral fourth interspace thoracotomy incision. Retraction of the pulmonary artery anteriorly allows dissection of the left main coronary artery and its bifurcation.

Selective coronary angiography in the patient illustrated (*A*) demonstrated significant involvement of the main left coronary artery and the origins of both the anterior descending branch and the circumflex artery. The lumen of the anterior descending artery beyond the arteriosclerotic plaque appeared suitable for an end-to-side anastomosis. Autogenous long saphenous vein is preferred for aorto-coronary by-pass graft. Surgical preparation should include the thigh in the field for the purpose of obtaining a generous segment of the long saphenous vein.

The operation is performed on cardiopulmonary by-pass. A short segment of the artery distal to the stenotic or occluded lesion is mobilized. Careful attention is required to avoid injury to side branches. The saphenous vein is prepared by ligation of the branches and dilation with heparin solution. An exclusion-type clamp is placed on the anterior wall of the aorta, and the distal end of the vein is anastomosed to the side of the ascending aorta (*B*). The other end of the vein is beveled by a longitudinal incision and an oblique end-to-side anastomosis carried out with the anterior descending branch of the left coronary artery. To obtain a quiet field for this anastomosis, hypothermia or electrically induced fibrillation may be employed.

PLATE 33

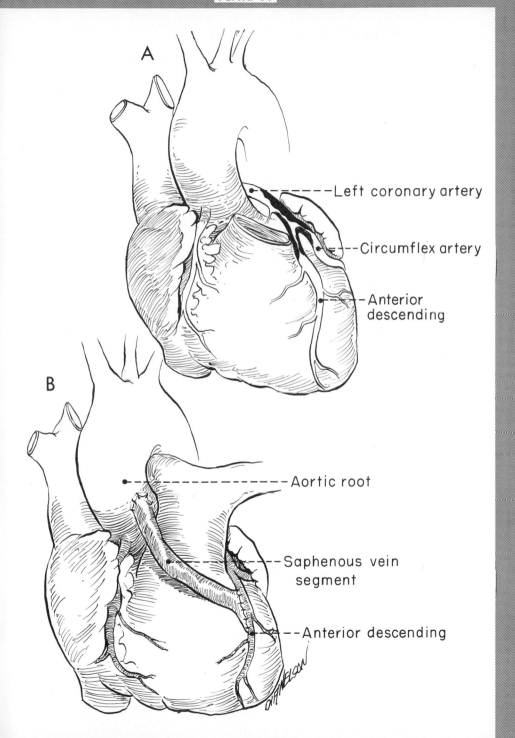

A

Left coronary artery

Circumflex artery

Anterior descending

B

Aortic root

Saphenous vein segment

Anterior descending

Severe localized occlusive disease in the right coronary artery in symptomatic patients offers an opportunity for direct arterial repair. Selective coronary arteriography affords the most practical way of assessing the surgical candidacy of an individual patient. Selection of the appropriate lesion for direct repair depends on an accurate anatomic localization of the obstruction and an appraisal of the distal arterial bed and its potential significance to the total coronary circulation.

Major obstruction in a dominant right coronary artery poses a serious threat to the patient's life and at the same time provides an excellent opportunity for direct approach. Various methods have been employed in an attempt to increase the blood flow through a diseased coronary artery. The selection of a suitable procedure depends greatly on the local findings and the proper interpretation of selective angiography. It must be remembered that failure to accomplish the surgical mission usually results in catastrophe.

Extracorporeal by-pass should be utilized routinely. Myocardial perfusion should be maintained throughout the procedure. One may augment coronary perfusion through a small catheter placed in the distal lumen of the artery while it is open and being repaired.

A median sternotomy provides satisfactory exposure (*A*). The right coronary artery should be carefully exposed. Heavy silk ligatures placed around the proximal and distal ends of the diseased segment facilitate retraction of the vessel and are useful for control of bleeding (*B*). A longitudinal incision in the diseased segment (*C*) exposes the atheromatous plaque (*D*). Endarterectomy should be attempted if the side branches do not exist or if they are completely occluded. Removal of the plaque (*E*) is particularly suited to a lesion that terminates within the confine of the arterial incision. Widening of the lumen can best be accomplished with an onlay patch graft of pericardium or a longitudinally incised segment of long saphenous vein (*F*).

In the majority of patients the atherosclerotic plaque extends distally, making the lesion unsuitable for endarterectomy. In these patients, gentle dilation of the arterial lumen distally and widening of the incised portion with an onlay vein patch graft provide the best result.

PLATE 34

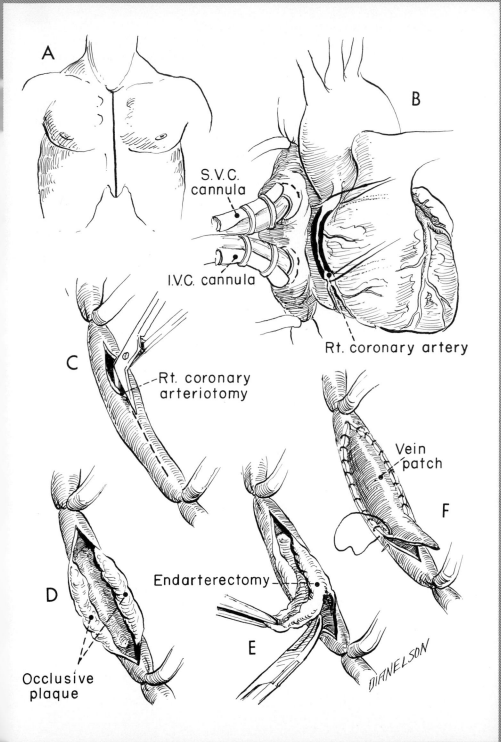

A

B

S.V.C.
cannula

I.V.C. cannula

Rt. coronary artery

C

Rt. coronary
arteriotomy

Vein
patch

F

D

Endarterectomy

Occlusive
plaque

E

DIANELSON

The left chest is elevated over a small sandbag, with the patient in an otherwise supine position. First, the left common femoral artery and vein are dissected free for subsequent cannulation. Then the left chest is entered through the fifth intercostal space by means of an anterolateral thoracotomy which is extended across the sternum without entering into the right pleural cavity (*A*). Not infrequently the pericardium is adherent to the aneurysm, and under these circumstances exposure is achieved only to the right ventricle and the right atrial appendage without manipulating the heart or the aneurysm.

The patient is heparinized and cannulation is carried out by inserting a catheter in the femoral artery and a large venous catheter into the inferior vena cava via the common femoral vein. A second venous catheter is passed into the right atrium through the right atrial appendage (*B*). It may be necessary to place the patient on partial by-pass, either for cardiac assist because of poor heart performance or to facilitate cannulation of the right atrium. When the patient is on by-pass, the pulmonary artery is clamped and the heart is made to fibrillate, using a sterile fibrillator unit (*B*). These maneuvers and the closure of the aortic valve as maintained by retrograde arterial flow prevent systemic embolism of fragments of clots from within the aneurysm. The heart and the aneurysm can now be dissected readily and the aneurysm entered, permitting evacuation of the mural thrombus (*C*). The sac is removed, leaving an adequate margin for closure (*D*). Care is taken not to injure the papillary muscles or major coronary branches.

Closure is carried out using interrupted horizontal everting mattress sutures reinforced with simple over-and-over sutures of nonabsorbable material (*E* and *F*). The pulmonary artery clamp is released, permitting some blood to fill the left-sided chambers and displace any air which may have been trapped in the heart. Interruption of fibrillation and restoration of cardiac contractions, either spontaneously or by electric countershock, aid in preventing air embolism. Often it is necessary to reinforce the closure by a strip of Teflon along each margin of the ventriculotomy.

PLATE 35

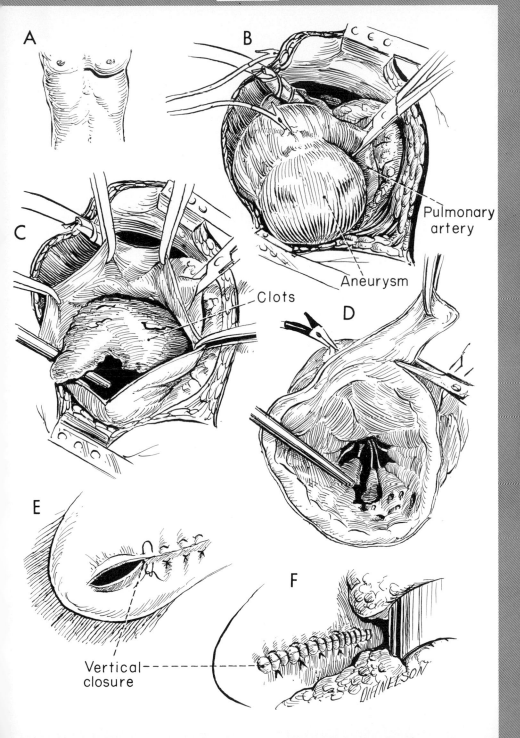

A

B

Pulmonary artery

Aneurysm

C

Clots

D

E

Vertical closure

F

D.H.NELSON

CHAPTER 7

Brachiocephalic Arterial Disease

THE HIGH INCIDENCE of occlusive disease of the carotid and subclavian arteries has been fully recognized in the past two decades. The effect of surgical removal of obstructing lesions in relieving symptoms of cerebral arterial insufficiency and in lowering the likelihood of stroke has also been appreciated. The carotid bifurcation is the commonest site of involvement. Occlusive disease here probably equals in frequency the rate of aortoiliac occlusive disease.

Carotid sinus atheroma produces symptoms of cerebral arterial insufficiency due to diminished cerebral perfusion caused by stenotic internal carotid arteries. These symptoms consist of lightheadedness and occasionally syncope, unilateral transient blurring, dimness of vision or blindness, and all varieties of sensory and motor dysfunction. Transient ischemic attacks (little stroke syndrome) can also be caused by emboli arising from an ulcerated atheromatous plaque at the carotid bifurcation.

Recognition of carotid bifurcation disease before a cerebral infarct or total obstruction of the cervical internal carotid artery occurs is most important if irreversible changes in the brain are to be avoided.

The presence of carotid bifurcation atheroma should be suspected in any patient who manifests transient ischemic attacks. The physical findings of a firm carotid bifurcation and a localized carotid bruit confirm the diagnosis.

The extent of internal carotid stenosis can only be estimated by carotid angiograms. A carotid compression test, ophthalmodynamometric studies, electroencephalography and brain scan are helpful but never reliably diagnostic. The absence of atheromatous involvement of the cervical internal carotid between the sinus and the base of the skull and the relative freedom of the common carotid artery proximal to the bifurcation emphasize the segmental nature of the lesion and make it amenable to surgical approach.

Carotid endarterectomy is indicated in severely stenotic lesions regardless of symptoms. The presence of an ulcerated carotid bifurcation plaque in patients with a clinical picture suggesting embolic cerebral lesions indicates the urgent need for surgical intervention. Carotid artery stenosis of less than 60 per cent in asymptomatic patients should be watched carefully by repeated physical examinations and carotid arteriograms. The rate of progress in the carotid sinus atheroma was evaluated in a large series of patients; it seemed to be related to severity of hypertension and the degree of local turbulence.

Patients with multiple lesions of brachiocephalic branches present challenging problems which require individualized surgical procedures. When a combination of internal carotid and vertebral artery stenoses exists, the carotid bifurcation endarterectomy should be attempted first. The vertebral artery lesion should also be corrected at a later date if symptoms persist.

Subclavian artery occlusion and vertebral subclavian steal syndrome deserve surgical attention only if the patient has symptoms of vertebral basilar insufficiency and/or upper extremity ischemia.

A percutaneous carotid arteriogram is most informative in visualizing the extracranial as well as the intracranial portion of the carotid system. This procedure does not require general anesthesia, and when it is performed with proper care, the incidence of neurologic complications should be below 1 per cent.

Bilateral percutaneous carotid arteriograms should be obtained in all patients and, with the use of Schonander or other comparable filming equipment, anteroposterior and lateral views should be evaluated with serial films. The site of needle puncture is most critical. The needle should never penetrate the atheroma at the level of the bifurcation. Neurologic complications of carotid arteriography relate most commonly to the dissection of the atheroma or the dislodgment of atheromatous debris.

Local infiltration of the skin (*A*) with Xylocaine or a comparable agent low in the neck along the medial border of the sternocleidomastoid muscle prepares the area for contrast injection (*B*). Penetration of the needle can be facilitated with a stab wound made with a size 11 scalpel. A Cournand needle is preferred whenever possible. A Teflon catheter needle is used when multiple injections in various neck positions are needed. It is of utmost importance to fill the tubing and needle with heparin solution to prevent clot formation and air introduction at the time of injection. Conray 60 is best tolerated by brain tissue; a 10 cc. injection in each carotid will suffice. Careful attention to the position of the arm avoids superimposition of shoulder and carotid bifurcation on a lateral view.

The radiographs *C* and *D* show carotid bifurcation disease. In *C* there is bilateral disease in a hypertensive individual with complete occlusion of the right internal carotid and 90 per cent stenosis of the left internal carotid artery. *D* shows an ulcerative carotid bifurcation atheroma. The presence of a niche, a fuzzy outline of the atheroma or contrast hang-up in the region of the atheroma suggest the probability of an ulcerated plaque.

PLATE 36

A

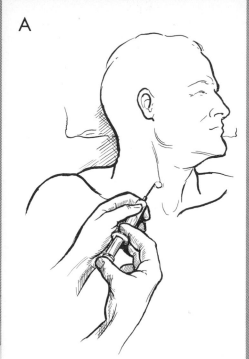

B

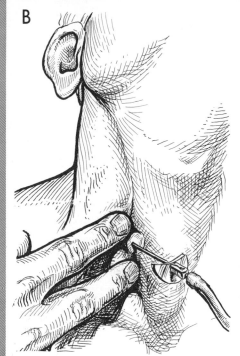

C

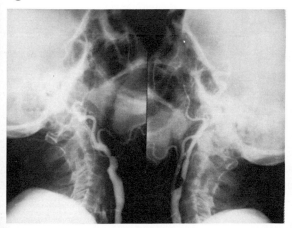

D

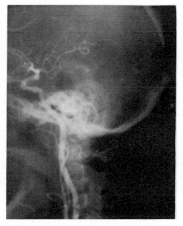

This procedure is indicated for severely stenotic lesions or for ulcerative plaques of the carotid bifurcation. Emergency surgery should be reserved for patients with frequent and progressive transient ischemic attacks in whom the internal carotid artery has a hair-line opening or an obvious ulcerative plaque. The disappearance of a carotid bruit and development of neurologic deficit in a patient with a known stenotic lesion suggests an emergency operation only if it can be done without delay.

Surgical intervention in patients with profound neurologic deficit and those with complete occlusion of the internal carotid artery has been disappointing in our experience.

General anesthesia is preferred whenever possible. Local anesthesia should be considered in extremely old individuals with severely altered cardiorespiratory reserve.

The carotid bifurcation is exposed through a longitudinal incision parallel to the anterior border of the sternocleidomastoid (*A*). The upper end of the incision should not extend beyond the angle of the jaw to avoid damage to the mandibular branch of the facial nerve. The facial vein and the midthyroid vein cross the carotid artery anteriorly and should be ligated and divided. Extreme care is required to avoid trauma to the hypoglossal nerve which crosses the bifurcation below the digastric muscle (*B*). The ansa of the hypoglossal nerve may be divided, if necessary, to obtain satisfactory exposure. Small veins also cross the internal carotid artery superiorly. These veins originate from the internal jugular vein and enter the wall of the pharynx. Control of bleeding from these veins may cause trauma to the hypoglossal nerve. The exposure of this area is indicated particularly in high-lying bifurcations. It is therefore appropriate to ligate and divide these veins before initiating the endarterectomy.

The superior thyroid branch of the external carotid artery should be encircled separately and preserved if possible. The dissection of the carotid bifurcation requires extreme care and gentleness to avoid dislodgment of the clot or atheromatous debris. The internal carotid artery is encircled with a tape, and the area beyond the atheromatous plaque is well exposed. Before proximal and distal cross-clamping of the arteries, 50 mg. of heparin is administered intravenously. *C* demonstrates the line of incision on the carotid bifurcation.

[Carotid endarterectomy *continued on page 116.*]

PLATE 37

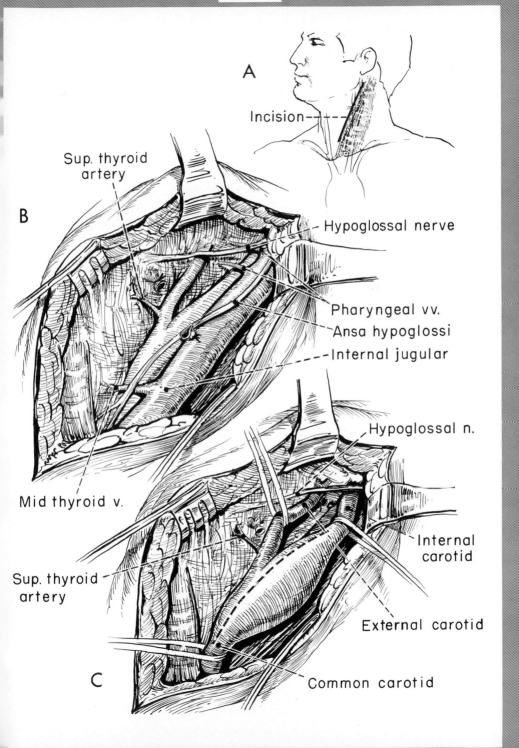

A

Incision

B

Sup. thyroid artery

Hypoglossal nerve

Pharyngeal vv.
Ansa hypoglossi
Internal jugular

Hypoglossal n.

Mid thyroid v.

Sup. thyroid artery

Internal carotid

External carotid

C

Common carotid

An intraluminal shunt consisting of a tapered polyvinyl flexible tube with olive-shaped tips has been routinely used. Specially devised clamps (Javid) secure the intraluminal tube in place (*D*).

The advantages of intraluminal shunting are many. Internal carotid flow is maintained. The need for haste is eliminated, assuring a careful endarterectomy and debridement of the arterial wall. The exposure to the upper end of the atheroma is improved by the presence of a loop outside the incision, which permits retraction at this level. The closure of the arteriotomy is also facilitated by the presence of the intraluminal stent, reducing the risk of stenosis of the internal carotid artery.

Certain precautions are necessary to minimize complications during the shunting procedure. The narrow end of the tube is introduced gently into the internal carotid artery after adequate exposure of the distal end of the atheroma. The small encircling clamp (Javid) is applied around the internal carotid artery well above the incision. The polyvinyl tube is then filled with blood by permitting retrograde flow and is pulled back to make certain that the tip is not blocked by lying against the wall of the artery. By unclamping the tube, one can estimate the quality of backflow. The larger end of the tube is then introduced into the common carotid artery to establish the cerebral flow. Extreme care is needed to avoid introduction of atheromatous particles into the tube, and particular attention is also needed to make certain no air bubbles remain in the system. The larger encircling clamp is then applied around the common carotid artery to establish the by-pass shunt.

Carotid endarterectomy should begin proximally by making a transverse incision of the intima at the lower end. The cleavage plane is quite apparent, and the separation of the intima from the artery wall can be accomplished with gentle retraction of the atheromatous plaque (*E*). The removal of the distal end of the atheroma, as demonstrated in *F*, is most essential. It is most important to leave the intima distally free from disease and well adherent to the outer layers.

Closure of the suture line is begun both proximally and distally (*G*). The intraluminal shunt is then removed in order to complete the suture line.

[Carotid endarterectomy *continued on page 118.*]

PLATE 37

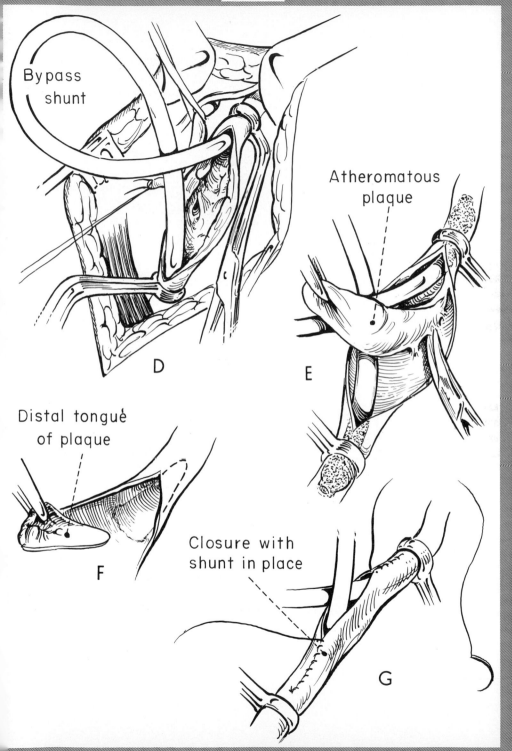

Bypass shunt

D

Atheromatous plaque

E

Distal tongue of plaque

F

Closure with shunt in place

G

The removal of the intraluminal shunt can be initiated by cross-clamping the tube or by pinching it with the fingers. The distal end should be pulled back gently; the blood flow from the internal carotid artery can be controlled by the use of a bulldog clamp or a comparable instrument (*H*). The proximal end of the by-pass tube is then removed, and the common carotid artery is cross-clamped to isolate the endarterectomized segment. The arterial lumen is irrigated with heparin solution to remove small fragments of atheromatous debris or residual clots. It is most important to remove all the remaining air bubbles by unclamping the internal carotid artery and permitting the retrograde flow to wash out the air bubbles through the opening in the incision before the suture line is completely sealed (*I*).

Restoration of flow should first be established into the external carotid artery by momentary clamping of the origin of the internal carotid artery (*J*). Again this is a precaution to prevent air bubbles or fragments remaining in the endarterectomized segment from entering into the more vital branch, the internal carotid artery. Restoration of flow to both internal and external carotid arteries is thus accomplished.

A patch of Dacron or of long saphenous vein has been used to enlarge the lumen of the internal carotid artery in rare instances in which the atheroma cannot be totally removed because of an unusual proximal or distal extension. A patch graft may also be useful in closures of the bifurcation area at any second operation upon it.

The use of protamine sulfate to neutralize the heparin effect has not been necessary in most patients.

The neck wound is drained routinely by a Penrose drain left in the dependent part of the incision. Anticoagulants are not employed in the postoperative period. Alterations in blood pressure in the immediate postoperative period should be treated aggressively.

A sudden development of neurologic deficit in a patient whose immediate course following carotid endarterectomy was considered uneventful should alert one to the possibility of thrombosis of the operative site. Immediate recognition of this complication and emergency re-exploration may avert catastrophic results.

PLATE 37

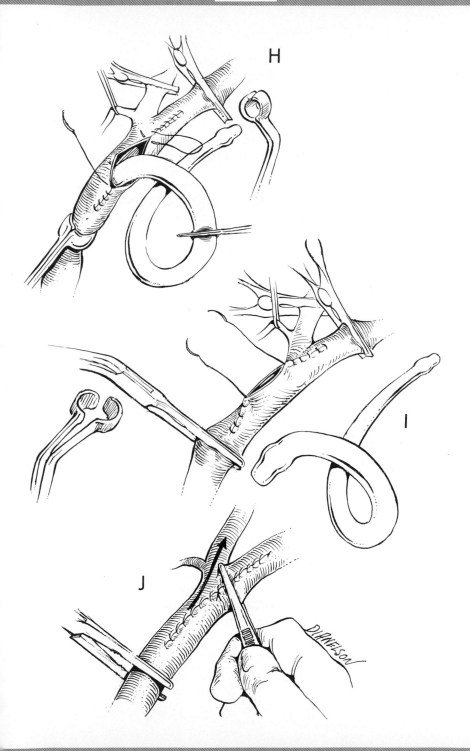

H

I

J

D.H.NELSON

Kinking of the internal carotid artery is commonly associated with atheromatous involvement of the carotid bifurcation and extreme tortuosity of the internal carotid artery beyond this level. Surgical intervention should be reserved for patients in whom clinical manifestations of carotid insufficiency correspond to the side of internal carotid artery kinking. Radiographic evidence of significant stenosis and often poststenotic dilatation can be demonstrated in the overwhelming majority of lesions. Production or aggravation of the symptoms by changing the position of the head and neck and disappearance or alteration of the neck bruit indicate strong likelihood of kinking of the carotid vessels. The mere presence of tortuosity is not an indication for surgical intervention.

Reimplantation of the internal carotid origin downward on the common carotid is corrective within the limits of any rigidity of the kinked segments. The carotid bifurcation is exposed exactly as described previously (Plate 37). Exposure of the tortuous internal carotid artery (*A*) requires careful dissection. The artery is often surrounded by fibrous bands, particularly at the level of the angulation. After adequate exposure is obtained, 50 mg. of heparin is administered intravenously. After proximal and distal cross-clamping, the origin of the internal carotid artery is transected, leaving a wide portion of the sinus attached to the internal carotid artery for reimplantation (*B*). A local endarterectomy of the mouth of the internal carotid artery should be accomplished if necessary by gently everting the cut end of the artery.

The by-pass shunt is then established by inserting the smaller end of the by-pass tube into the internal carotid artery and securing it in place by an encircling clamp (*C*). The proximal end of the by-pass tube is inserted into an incision in the common carotid artery at a level estimated to be the proper location of the origin of the internal carotid artery. Depending on the length of the internal carotid artery and the location of the kink, the surgeon may choose the anterior or the posterior wall of the common carotid artery for the reimplantation of the origin of the internal carotid artery. The posterior suture line is completed first, as shown in *D*, and partial closure of the anterior suture line can be accomplished before removal of the intraluminal shunt. *E* illustrates the completed procedure, which has eliminated the tortuosity and kinking of the artery.

PLATE 38

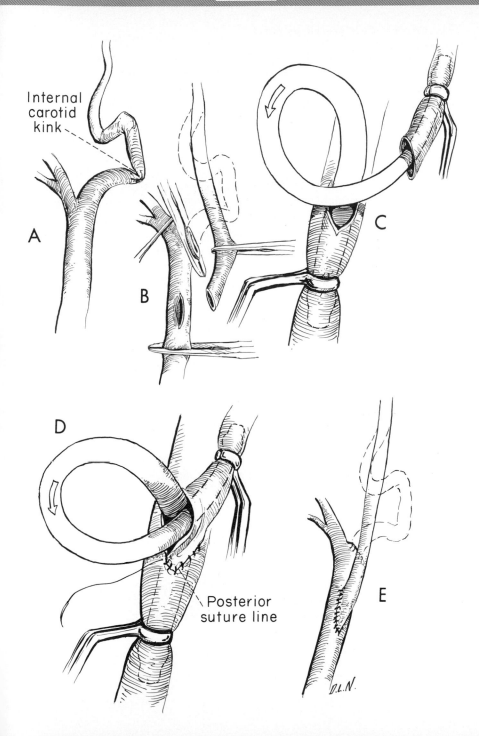

Internal carotid kink

A

B

C

D

Posterior suture line

E

D.L.N.

Establishment of a carotid subclavian by-pass graft in the neck is useful in the management of complete occlusion of the subclavian artery or of complete common carotid occlusion with patency of the carotid bifurcation. Occasionally there is a combination of internal carotid artery stenosis and complete occlusion of the proximal portion of the subclavian artery. Here both carotid endarterectomy and a carotid subclavian by-pass can be accomplished to restore flow to both the internal carotid artery and the subclavian artery simultaneously. The operative procedure is similar for the above-mentioned lesions, with the possible exception that in a patient with a normal carotid artery one may wish to anastomose the graft to the common carotid artery below the bifurcation somewhere at the base of the neck. The other steps of the procedure remain similar, and it is appropriate, therefore, to illustrate the combined carotid endarterectomy and carotid subclavian by-pass in this plate.

Exposure to the carotid bifurcation and the cervical portion of the subclavian artery can be accomplished through two separate neck incisions (*A*). One incision is made parallel to the sternocleidomastoid similar to the incision discussed previously for carotid bifurcation endarterectomy (Plate 37). The other incision is made above the clavicle in a transverse fashion for exposure of the subclavian artery.

This exposure is obtained by transection of the scalenus anticus muscle and retraction of the phrenic nerve medially; particular care is necessary in the dissection of the subclavian artery to avoid entrance into the pleural space. *B* demonstrates the exposure of the subclavian artery and shows an exclusion clamp in place, with a completed end-to-side anastomosis between an 8 mm. Dacron graft and the subclavian artery. The patient is given 50 mg. of heparin intravenously before the application of the clamp. The Dacron graft has been preclotted before administration of the heparin.

The exposure of the carotid bifurcation is shown in *C*. The internal shunt is employed routinely and the carotid endarterectomy is carried out in the manner discussed in Plate 37 and illustrated in *D*. The atheromatous plaque often extends distally over the normal intima as a tonguelike projection, requiring careful separation of the plaque from the wall (*E*).

[Carotid subclavian by-pass *continued on page 124.*]

PLATE 39

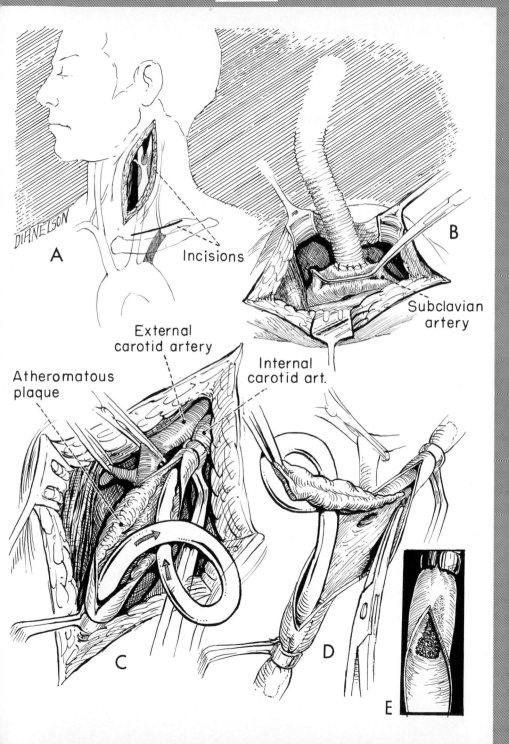

DIHNELSON

A

Incisions

B

Subclavian artery

External carotid artery

Internal carotid art.

Atheromatous plaque

C

D

E

A tunnel is constructed underneath a flap of the skin between the two incisions (*F*), preferably deep to the sternocleidomastoid, and the 8 mm. Dacron graft is passed through the tunnel to be anastomosed to the carotid bifurcation. The anastomosis can be accomplished at the lower end of the incision, provided the internal carotid artery is a large vessel and the repair can be accomplished without compromising the size of the lumen (*G*). In patients with small common or internal carotid arteries it may be preferable to cut the end of the graft in an oblique fashion (*H*) and suture the beveled end to the entire carotid bifurcation incision. The posterior suture line is completed first and, after partial closure of the anterior suture line (*I*), the shunt is removed. The anastomosis is then completed.

It is of vital importance to clear the graft of clots and to remove the air bubbles to avoid catastrophic complications of emboli. The subclavian clamp is first removed to fill the entire graft with blood prior to completion of the suture line, and the graft is compressed between the operator's fingers to avoid undue blood loss. With the graft compressed, the clamp on the internal carotid artery is released to determine the retrograde flow and to empty air bubbles from the carotid system. After completion of the anastomosis, the flow is first established into the external carotid and the subclavian arteries by compressing the internal carotid artery with thumb forceps (*J*), again to avoid air embolization, and then the flow is established into the internal carotid artery by unclamping this vessel. In this manner the arterial flow is restored to the carotid system as well as to the subclavian artery.

This procedure is preferred to transthoracic aorto-subclavian by-pass whenever feasible. In patients with extensive involvement of the common carotid artery and complete occlusion of the subclavian artery, a transthoracic approach for restoration of subclavian flow may be chosen, and at a later stage a by-pass graft in the neck between the subclavian artery and the carotid bifurcation may be accomplished if indicated.

PLATE 39

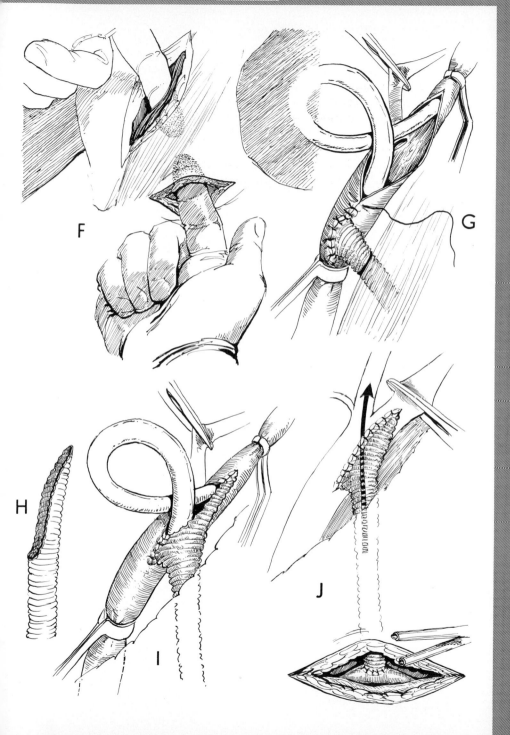

F

G

H

I

J

Occasionally the subclavian artery occlusion is not confined to the proximal portion of this artery but extends beyond the origin of the vertebral artery and thyrocervical trunk. The atheromatous involvement of the cervical portion of the subclavian artery precludes the possibility of a carotid-subclavian by-pass in the neck or an aorto-subclavian by-pass transthoracically. These patients often experience severe upper extremity claudication or rest pain, necessitating restoration of flow. The procedure illustrated here has been successful in a number of patients, using a Dacron prosthesis or a long saphenous vein graft.

The patient is positioned on the operating table with the arm abducted and suspended overhead to a screen (*A*). The patient is in a 45-degree lateral position. The goal of the operation is to establish a by-pass between the ascending aorta and the right axillary artery in patients with right subclavian artery occlusion (*B*). A similar procedure can be done on the left side by originating the graft from the descending aorta.

Exposure of the axillary artery can be accomplished through a transverse incision in the axilla. Careful dissection of the artery at this level should be done first to determine the patency of the vessel and the feasibility of performing an aorto-axillary by-pass graft.

The ascending aorta is exposed through a right submammary fourth intercostal space incision. The pericardium is incised longitudinally to expose the ascending aorta (*C*). A portion of the ascending aorta is excluded with a laterally applied clamp, and an end-to-side anastomosis between an 8 mm. preclotted Dacron graft and a longitudinal incision in the excluded portion of the aorta is accomplished.

The graft is passed along the apex of the thoracic cage and is brought out into the axillary wound through a tunnel created in the first interspace. End-to-side anastomosis between the graft and the side of the axillary artery is then accomplished (*D*). The graft usually takes a gentle curve in the thoracic cage and can be covered by the pleura if desired. Removal of the sympathetic chain from the first to fifth ganglion is desirable and does not add greatly to the length of the procedure.

In patients with a thin-walled axillary artery, a vein by-pass graft may be preferable. Long saphenous vein by-pass grafts have been implanted in a number of patients with excellent long-term results.

PLATE 40

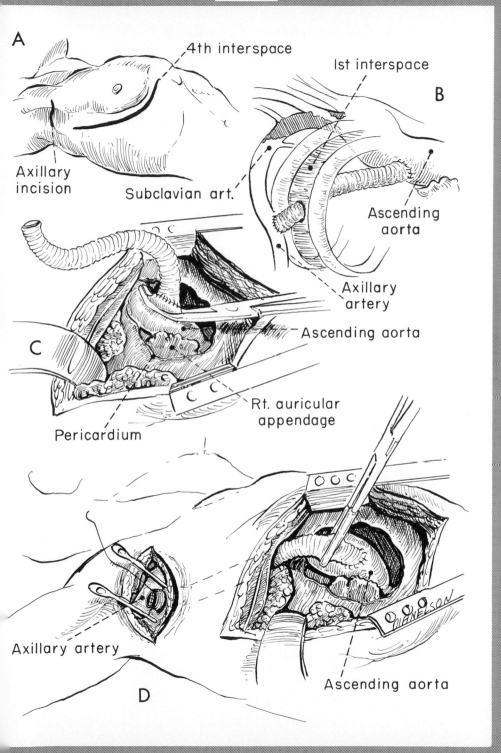

A
4th interspace
1st interspace
B
Axillary incision
Subclavian art.
Ascending aorta
Axillary artery
Ascending aorta
C
Rt. auricular appendage
Pericardium
Axillary artery
D
Ascending aorta

A stenotic lesion of the origin of the vertebral artery can best be repaired by a patch graft. There is often involvement of the subclavian artery as well as the vertebral artery, and the lesion does not lend itself to a local endarterectomy. The procedure which provides the most reliable restoration of flow is one in which the subclavian artery and the vertebral artery at its origin are opened in continuity. Wide patency of the vessel is assured by the use of a generous patch graft of flat vein wall obtained from the long saphenous system. Temporary intraluminal shunting is most difficult and has not been employed.

To expose the vertebral artery origin, a supraclavicular incision is made (*A*), extending from the sternal notch for a distance of 3 – 4 in. laterally. The incision is made parallel to the clavicle and, after division of the platysma muscle in the direction of the skin incision, the clavicular attachment of the sternocleidomastoid muscle is transected to get sufficient exposure medially. The phrenic nerve is identified, retracted medially and left intact. The transverse cervical artery is divided. The next step is transection of the scalenus anticus muscle. The bleeding in the muscle substance is controlled by cautery, and the subclavian artery is exposed immediately underneath the muscle. Division of the thyrocervical trunk and the internal mammary artery is required for adequate mobilization of the subclavian artery in order to expose the vertebral origin. *B* demonstrates satisfactory exposure of the subclavian artery and vertebral origin.

After the patient has received 50 mg. of heparin intravenously, proximal and distal cross-clamping is accomplished. The line of incision extends from the subclavian artery into the origin of the vertebral artery and to a distance about 1 cm. beyond the origin. A convenient method of gaining gentle traction on the vessel is to use a Cooley vascular clamp proximal to the origin of the vertebral artery, passing it from behind the vertebral junction. The length of the incision in the vertebral artery depends on the length of the segment of vertebral artery involved. An elliptic patch of saphenous vein is then implanted to provide a broad vertebral artery origin (*C*).

PLATE 41

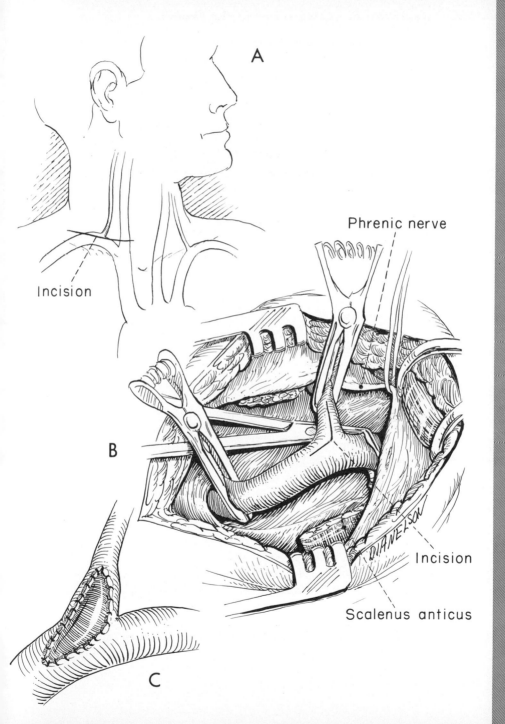

A

Incision

Phrenic nerve

B

DIANELSON

Incision

Scalenus anticus

C

Interference with blood supply to the upper extremity, other than that caused by arteriosclerotic lesions of the subclavian and axillary arteries, is produced by structural abnormalities in the musculoskeletal route taken by the blood vessels and nerves through the shoulder girdle. The subclavian artery and the brachial plexus may be compressed anteriorly by a prominent bony projection at the level of the scalenus anticus muscle attachment to the first rib or by a callus from a fractured clavicle. Cervical rib or fibrous bands attaching this anomalous bony appendage to the first rib compress the neurovascular bundle from behind. An abnormal relationship between the first rib and the clavical causes squeezing of the subclavian artery, subclavian vein and brachial plexus as they traverse the narrowed costoclavicular space.

Often it is difficult to appreciate the exact location of the neurovascular compression in the neck and shoulder. Occasionally a poststenotic dilatation in the subclavian artery can be detected by palpation of the neck indicating a compression by a band from the cervical rib attachment to the first rib. The presence of a bruit over the subclavian artery in a young individual with typical paresthesia along the inner aspect of the arm and forearm may give a clue to the presence of compressive syndrome. The appearance of an audible bruit by the change of arm position or the abolition of pulse in the arm are confirmative diagnostic signs. In patients with compression of the neurovascular bundle at the costoclavicular angle, upper extremity vein engorgement accompanies alteration in pulse. Traction of the upper extremity downward, the assumption of attention position or bracing of the shoulder often aggravate the symptoms. Subclavian arteriography adds information if an atheromatous lesion has developed at the site of arterial impingement or if aneurysmal dilatation distal to the compression area is present.

The symptoms of neurovascular compression are similar, regardless of the cause. The compression is usually intermittent, and the symptoms are present at first only during periods of effective impingement, usually when the patient assumes a recumbent position in the case of a cervical rib or when the individual carries heavy objects in the case of costoclavicular compression. After some time, the nerve and artery sustain some degree of permanent damage. Pain, paresthesia and muscle atrophy may then follow because of nerve damage, while arterial insufficiency leads to numbness of the fingers and upper extremity claudication. Occasionally patients experience necrosis of the finger-tips and ischemic neuritis. The factor of peripheral arterial constriction is important in the development of severe ischemic changes. Another feature of these conditions is suggested by the occasional presence of occlusive lesions in the brachial artery. The distal obstructions are probably embolic, the embolus having arisen from a thrombus formed at the level of arterial impingement. The two elements of arterial constriction and peripheral emboli account for severe ischemia in lesions of the subclavian artery, a region thought to be extraordinarily well protected by available collateral arteries.

When a situation productive of vascular or nerve compression is demonstrated, its early surgical correction is indicated as prophylaxis against permanent damage to the compressed structures. Appropriate surgical procedures for each type of lesion are described in the following pages. In every case it is important to investigate the adequacy of the size of the total route taken by vessels and nerves throughout the cervicoaxillary tunnel. The artery may easily be encroached upon by more than a single abnormality, and after the scalenus anticus compression has been effectively relieved, palpation of the route is indicated to determine the need for resection of a portion of the first rib.

Anomalous development of the costal tubercle of the seventh cervical vertebra may occasionally become a sizable bony projection. The neurovascular compression is caused by the cervical rib itself or by a fibrous attachment that connects this bony structure to the first rib. *A* demonstrates the usual angulation of the neurovascular bundle, which often involves the lower trunk of the brachial plexus, producing neurologic disturbances along the ulnar pathway. Indication for surgery is based on the presence of a cervical rib on x-ray studies, local findings of the bony prominence in the neck, the detection of a bruit over the subclavian artery on abduction of the arm to a 90-degree level and alteration of the wrist pulses, denoting arterial compression. The symptoms are usually typical, in that the patient experiences intermittent attacks of paresthesia and pain along the ulnar distribution. Patients often wake up with neurologic symptoms and can relieve the discomfort by a change in arm position. The mere presence of a cervical rib does not indicate the need for surgical intervention.

Approach to the cervical rib can be obtained through a transverse incision in the supraclavicular region. The clavicular attachments of the sternocleidomastoid muscle are transected, and the transverse cervical artery is ligated and divided. The phrenic nerve which crosses the scalenus anticus muscle and traverses along the medial border of the lower attachment of this muscle is preserved (*B* and *C*). The muscle fibers are then cut, and the bleeding from the muscle substance is controlled with suture ligature or cautery. The subclavian artery is exposed immediately behind the scalenus anticus muscle. The space between the cervical rib and the brachial plexus is developed by blunt dissection, and with gentle retraction of the neurovascular bundle medially, the cervical rib and its attachment are exposed (*D*). The fibrous band is totally excised, and the bony projection is removed with a rongeur until the compression from behind is completely eliminated. *E* shows the relationship of the cervical rib, the scalenus anticus and the neurovascular bundle.

Occasionally chronic impingement of the subclavian artery may produce poststenotic dilatation or aneurysm formation in this vessel, requiring excision of the diseased portion and replacement by a prosthesis. A segment of long saphenous vein of adequate size has been used with satisfactory results.

PLATE 42

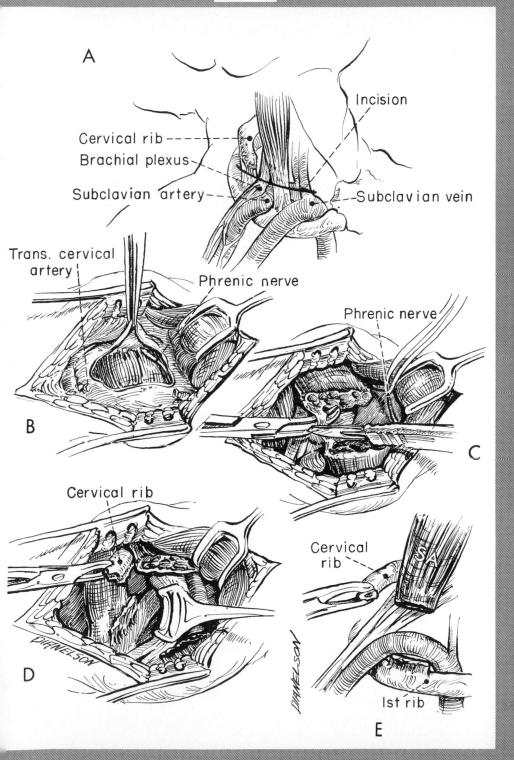

A

Cervical rib

Brachial plexus

Subclavian artery

Incision

Subclavian vein

Trans. cervical
artery

Phrenic nerve

Phrenic nerve

B

C

Cervical rib

Cervical
rib

D

1st rib

E

The compression in the costoclavicular triangle affects both the subclavian artery and vein in addition to the brachial plexus (*A*). The cause of this abnormal relationship is not clear, but the elevation of the first rib, abnormality of the contour of the clavicle, hypertrophy of the subclavian muscle and atrophy of the shoulder muscles producing drooping of the shoulder are factors involved. Treatment consists of sectioning the scalenus anticus muscle and a generous resection of the first rib, including the periosteum, to enable the neurovascular bundle to assume a lower position free from compression. Removal of the clavicle should never be considered.

The exposure to the first rib can be accomplished through the neck or through an axillary incision. The advantage of the cervical approach is that one can examine other areas of compression in the neck and remove compressive bands, if present. A transverse incision above and parallel to the clavicle provides adequate exposure after transection of the clavicular attachments of the sternocleidomastoid and transection of the scalenus anticus muscle (*A*). The subclavian artery is then dissected free and encircled with a cord tape (*B*). The space between the clavicle and the first rib can be explored by the index finger and the area of compression determined (*C*).

The approach to the first rib is best accomplished by retraction of the brachial plexus laterally to provide maximum protection and to avoid trauma to the nerve fibers (*D*). Removal of the first rib is best accomplished by the use of a rongeur. Retraction of the subclavian artery medially or laterally (*E*) will improve the exposure for removing a generous portion of the first rib and will provide adequate room for the passage of the neurovascular bundle. The excision of the rib must include the periosteum so that bony regeneration will not take place.

A transaxillary approach should be considered in patients in whom the absolute diagnosis of costoclavicular compression syndrome is confirmed by angiography. Resection of a portion of the first rib can be accomplished through a transverse axillary incision. The patient is placed in a 90-degree lateral position with the arm abducted and suspended overhead. Retraction of the latissimus dorsi and pectoralis muscles provides adequate exposure to the first rib and the neurovascular bundle.

PLATE 43

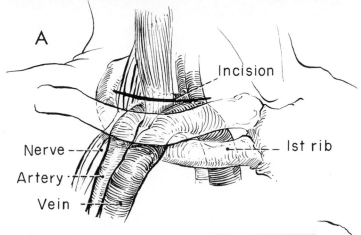

A

Incision

Nerve

Artery

Vein

Ist rib

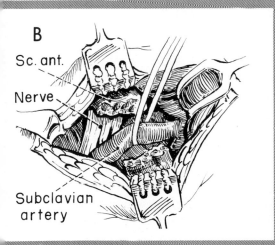

B

Sc. ant.

Nerve

Subclavian
artery

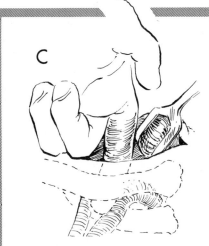

C

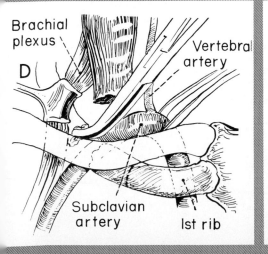

Brachial
plexus

Vertebra
artery

D

Subclavian
artery

Ist rib

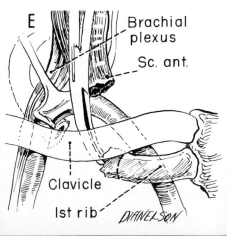

E

Brachial
plexus

Sc. ant.

Clavicle

Ist rib

DIFINELSON

CHAPTER **8**

Hypertension Due
to Renovascular Disease

HYPERTENSION occurs in the presence of lesions which disturb renal artery flow either because of the altered volume of flow or because of changes in the pulse-pressure curve. As a consequence of the pathologic hemodynamics, a very potent vasopressor substance enters the circulation. Surgical therapy often succeeds in its aims to restore normal renal hemodynamics and to relieve the hypertension. The possibility of a disturbance in the anatomy of the renal vasculature should be a paramount consideration in the evaluation of patients with arterial hypertension.

Segmental arteriosclerosis is the most frequent cause of renal artery stenosis. Less common lesions which disturb renal flow include idiopathic congenital stenosis, fibromuscular hyperplasia, nonspecific arteritis, syphilitic arteritis, compression of the renal artery by malignancy or aneurysm and the renal arterial narrowing associated with abdominal coarctation. No age group is exempt from this etiology of hypertension. Suspicion of its presence should be particularly aroused by the following clues.

1. Significant hypertension in children or young adults.

2. Hypertension of abrupt onset.

3. Elevated blood pressure in patients with a history suggestive of renovascular accident, such as embolism.

4. Severe hypertension rapidly progressing to malignant phase.

5. Mild hypertension that suddenly becomes severe.

6. Malignant hypertension in the older age group.

7. Hypertension in the patient with known arteriosclerotic disease elsewhere in the vascular system.

The physical findings in patients with renal artery stenosis are seldom diagnostic. Routine investigation of the urinary tract usually gives negative results. The diagnosis, therefore, is established only by the use of special diagnostic techniques. These include: intravenous pyelography with special timing of the x-ray exposures, split tests of kidney function carried out either by retrograde ureteral catheterization or by a radioisotope renogram, the angiotensin infusion test, assays of renal venous blood for renin, and renal arteriography.

During intravenous pyelography, film exposures are obtained at intervals between 30 seconds and two minutes after injection of the excretory dye. These early films will often show a delay of excretion by the kidney with arterial involvement as compared to the normal kidney, whereas in the customary five-minute film the concentration of dye in the renal pelves as seen by x-ray will be equal. The kidney on the side of the arterial stenosis will usually be smaller.

Interpretation of the split renal function test using ureteral catheterization depends on the fact that electrolyte excretion of the kidney is depressed in renal ischemia. In particular, less sodium is excreted and the total volume output of the involved kidney per unit of time is also diminished. The radioisotope renogram consists of the study of the curve of radioactivity over each kidney after injection of tagged substances which are excreted by the kidney. The split tests of kidney function are valuable in comparing the two sides, but the results may be misleading or difficult to evaluate when bilateral disease is present.

The relatively simple angiotensin infusion test depends on the fact that the patient with circulating angiotensin excess from his ischemic kidney will have a lesser hypertensive response to the administration of exogenous synthetic angiotensin. Bioassay of venous renin activity may be of value in special situations, although there are difficulties inherent in these studies.

Aortography for visualization of the renal arteries is a prerequisite to surgery, not only because it provides anatomic proof of the presence of the arterial lesion but also because it delineates the pathology from the standpoint of feasibility of repair.

Two techniques are used for visualizing the renal arteries. One is the translumbar percutaneous puncture of the aorta, and the second is a retrograde method in which a catheter is passed upward from the femoral artery until its tip lies in the region of the renal artery origins.

The translumbar method of aortography is described on page 34. This method of renal artery visualization is used principally in adults who have distal aneurysmal or occlusive disease of the aorta and its branches in addition to suspect renal vascular disease. The needle is placed in such a fashion as to be at a level slightly higher than that for routine translumbar aortography, and 20–25 ml. of contrast medium is injected. *A* shows the course of the needle into the aorta with the patient sedated and lying on his abdomen. The accompanying radiograph shows marked stenosis of the right renal artery with the poststenotic dilatation.

More commonly, renal arteriography is performed via the transfemoral catheter. This is the technique of choice and is used in all instances except those in which there is peripheral vascular disease distal to the renal arteries. A patient with iliac artery stenosis or superficial artery occlusion, for example, should not have retrograde femoral artery catheterization. The catheter is introduced in the artery percutaneous over a needle, except in children in whom direct exposure of the artery via a small skin incision may be preferable. The catheter then may be positioned freely in the aorta and the tip so placed as to permit injection in the immediate vicinity of the renal arteries. *B* shows the position of the catheter in the study of a patient with right renal artery stenosis. The accompanying radiograph shows the lesion of fibromuscular hyperplasia involving the lateral third of the renal artery. The patient, a young female, later had resection of the involved artery with end-to-end anastomosis and cure of her hypertension.

Regardless of the method of aortography, it is desirable to use x-ray equipment capable of making multiple exposures during the injection of contrast medium. By reviewing multiple films with the dye passing serially through the vessels being studied, maximum information can be gained.

PLATE 44

A

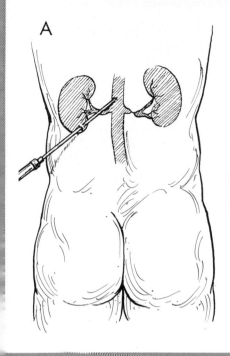

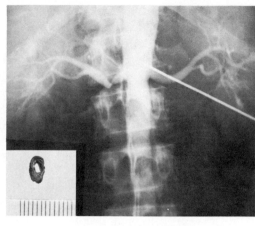

B

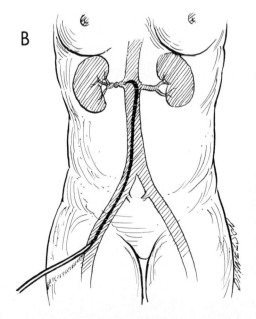

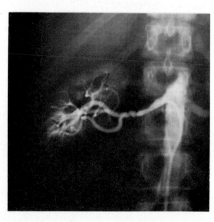

Transperitoneal vertical incisions are most often used, as they facilitate exposure of both renal arterial origins and permit convenient management of coexisting lesions of the abdominal aorta and its pelvic branches. Subcostal or transverse incisions are sometimes used when lesions are located in the middle or lateral third of the renal artery.

In *A*, a paramedian incision has been used to open the abdomen. The transverse colon and the omentum have been brought up out of the abdomen superiorly, while loops of small intestine have been retracted to the right. The incision in the posterior parietal peritoneum has been made longitudinally just to the right of the inferior mesenteric vein. This incision is carried upward through the ligament of Treitz to as high a level as possible, often exposing the inferior margin of the pancreas. The left renal vein and the vena cava are freed from the surrounding tissue and may be retracted safely, using a Penrose drain passed about each vessel (*B*). With these veins retracted, a considerable length of the right renal artery (*C*) may be exposed. Exposure of the left renal artery offers comparatively little difficulty. Palpation of the arteries serves generally to outline the stenosing lesion and to determine its extent. The true severity of the lesion can be determined only by direct pressure measurement of aorta and distal renal artery.

Localized stenosis occurring 1–2 cm. from the renal artery origin may be managed by resection of the stenosed area. Oblique lines of transection (*D*) are used in order to produce a long oblique nonconstricting anastomosis (*E*). Vessel length is adequate for sacrifice of 10–15 mm. of vessel in virtually every case.

A localized stenosis at the origin of the renal artery (*F*) can be corrected by transplantation of the artery to a slightly lower point on the aorta if the latter is thin and reasonably normal. The new connection is made to an area of the aortic wall isolated in a curved clamp (*G*) or more often to a portion of the aortic wall isolated by cross-clamping above and below the aortotomy. The end-to-side anastomosis (*H*) is made with either interrupted or continuous sutures or a combination of the two techniques.

The longer area of stenosis shown in the lower figure of *F* is unsuitable for these techniques and requires a grafting procedure.

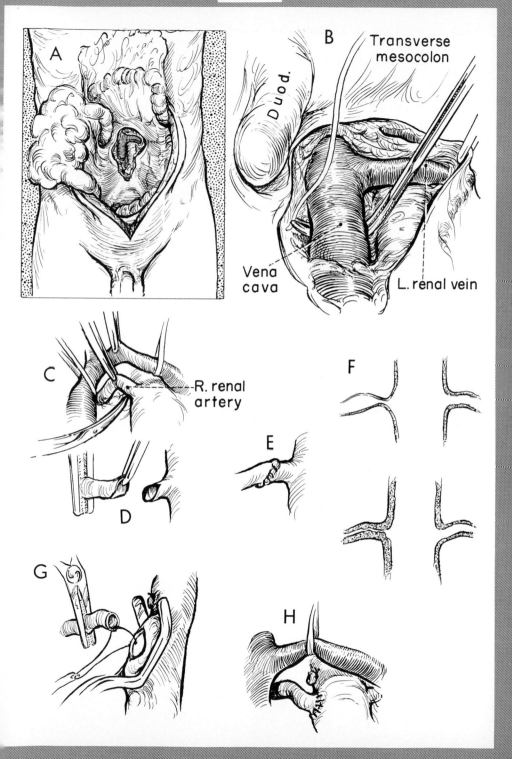

PLATE 45

B. Transverse mesocolon

Duod.

Vena cava

L. renal vein

C. R. renal artery

Most reconstructions of the renal arteries involve the use of a by-pass prosthetic or autogenous vein graft. The arteriosclerotic lesion in the proximal artery (*A*) is conveniently treated by this method. As shown in Plate 46, most often we utilize a prosthetic graft (8 mm. in diameter), but on occasion we have used a saphenous vein and even very exceptionally an internal iliac artery.

After the transperitoneal incision is made, the retroperitoneal tissues are opened and the aorta and both of the renal arteries are exposed. The renal arteries are inspected and the presence of an obstruction confirmed. Pressure determinations are made and kidney biopsies performed.

The aorta is isolated just distal to the renal arteries and its wall carefully palpated. If the wall is thin and suitable for end-to-side anastomosis, this portion of the aorta is isolated (*B*) and a short length of preclotted 8 mm. diameter graft is anastomosed end-to-side, using a synthetic suture. Heparin should be given either into the distal aortic segment or systemically prior to cross-clamping to prevent intraluminal clotting. After the anastomosis is complete, a clamp is placed on the graft and the aortic clamps may be removed.

The renal artery is isolated between noncrushing clamps and opened distal to its narrowed portion (*C*). An end-to-side anastomosis is performed between it and the graft. It is important that dilute heparin solution be placed in the distal renal artery prior to cross-clamping to prevent thrombosis in the small arterial branches at the kidney hilus. Delicate handling and fine synthetic sutures must be used because the renal artery is often fragile and subject to tearing. Renal artery cross-clamping is tolerated for 15–30 minutes without hypothermia. *D* shows the completed anastomosis with the functioning graft in place.

If both renal arteries require reconstruction, a bifurcation graft of small caliber may be anastomosed to the aorta (*E*) and the respective limbs anastomosed to the renal arteries. When an abdominal aortic aneurysm exists or aortoiliac occlusive disease requires reconstruction, the by-pass graft may be sutured as a side arm of the aortic prosthesis (*F*). If the pathology in the renal artery extends out to the first major division, it may be technically preferable to perform an end-to-end anastomosis between graft and renal artery, as shown in *G*.

PLATE 46

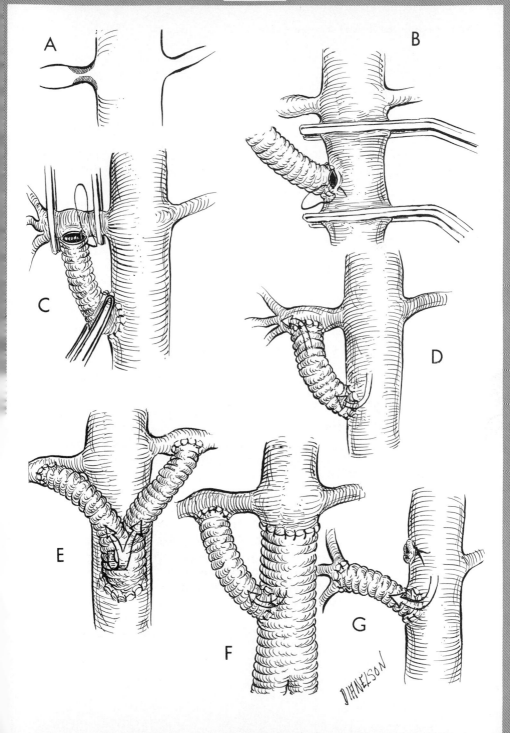

A   B   C   D   E   F   G

DHNELSON

The most common cause of renovascular hypertension is renal artery stenosis, and the most frequent reason for the surgeon to operate on the renal arteries is to relieve this condition. There are, however, other lesions of the renal arteries requiring surgical treatment which may be associated with blood pressure elevation. These include renal artery aneurysm, renal arteriovenous fistula and renal arterial thrombosis or embolism. Whether hypertension is present or not, operation may be indicated to correct these lesions.

Renal artery embolus most often will occur as a consequence of heart disease. An uncommon etiology is shown in Plate 47, *A*. In this patient the right renal artery became blocked by an embolus during retrograde aortography performed to confirm the presence of a suprarenal pheochromocytoma. Renal artery thrombosis will occur in a vessel previously strictured by disease. Hypertension may occur if the kidney is not infarcted but rather rendered totally or in part ischemic.

The aortogram in *A* demonstrates occlusion of the right renal artery by an embolus at its first major division. Through a transperitoneal flank incision, the right kidney with its suprarenal and hilar structures was exposed. After removal of a pheochromocytoma, the renal artery was clamped (*B*), a transverse arteriotomy performed and the embolus removed with the assistance of a small balloon-tipped catheter. The vessel was repaired without producing stricture and normal flow was permitted into the kidney (*C*).

Renal artery aneurysms may be congenital or acquired. The acquired ones are principally caused by arteriosclerosis. Such aneurysms may produce the Goldblatt phenomenon, and they have a distinct tendency to rupture. An aneurysm involving the main renal artery, as seen on the arteriogram *D*, can be resected with preservation of the kidney. The main renal artery and the secondary divisions are isolated as shown in *E* after heparinization of the isolated and interrupted local circulation. Removal of the aneurysm is then carried out, with end-to-end reconstruction of the renal artery (*F*).

Renal arteriovenous fistulae are principally due to penetrating injuries, although they may also be congenital or caused by neoplasm. Hypertension almost always results. Invariably nephrectomy is required to interrupt the fistula.

PLATE 47

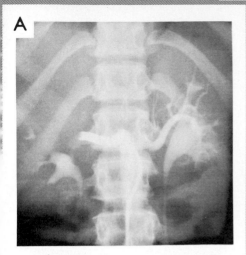

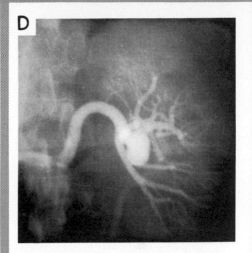

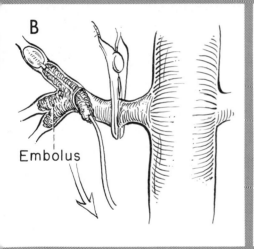

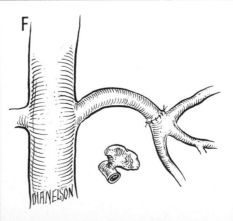

Embolus

Aneurysm

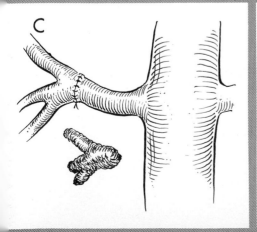

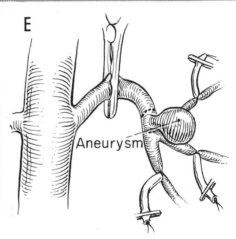

CHAPTER 9

Arterial Aneurysm

TRUE ANEURYSMAL dilatation involving all layers of the vessel wall occurs in an artery when its elastic properties are destroyed by infection or degenerative processes, or when the lateral stress on the arterial wall is increased by some abnormality in flow, such as that which occurs distal to a constriction or stenosis. The resulting dilatation is given the descriptive name of saccular aneurysm or fusiform aneurysm. A saccular aneurysm, being one which arises from a relatively small area of the artery wall, is much more likely to be produced by syphilitic infection, whereas a fusiform aneurysm, which involves weakening of the entire circumference of the vessel wall, is principally produced by arteriosclerosis. Pyogenic infections of a blood vessel wall result from lodgment of an infected embolus. Aneurysms formed on this basis are termed mycotic aneurysms. They usually have peripheral locations in medium- and small-sized vessels.

An example of poststenotic aneurysm is the dilatation, sometimes to large size, seen just distal to a coarctation of the thoracic aorta. Another example of poststenotic aneurysm formation is occasionally seen in the abdominal aorta, where resection of an infrarenal aortic aneurysm may show the aorta just proximal to the aneurysm to be the site of segmental stenosis.

Dissecting aneurysms, which are also called dissecting hematomas, are structurally quite different from true aneurysm. These lesions develop when a tear in the intima and internal layers of the media allows blood to escape into a potential or already developed layer of separation within the media of the vessel. The outer coats, no longer able to support the pressure of blood flow, expand to aneurysmal proportions. This lesion, often one of acute

146

onset, involves one of at least three predisposing factors. One is hypertension. Dissecting aneurysm may occur in hypertensive patients whose arteries are not the site of any other severe pathologic change. A second factor is ulcerative atherosclerosis. In examples of this, the dissection is apparently based on escape of blood into the vessel wall through the edge of an atherosclerotic plaque. These lesions are sometimes well localized, extending only modest distances in the dissecting layer above and below the point of internal defect. Finally, the most disastrous form occurs in individuals having pre-existing degenerative changes within the media of the type often associated with other anomalies of Marfan's syndrome. The dissection in these cases rarely remains localized for long, although exceptions are seen and present as candidates for surgical reconstruction.

The surgical treatment of a variety of aneurysms is depicted in Plates 49 to 63 according to the locations in which they occur. Of greatest importance in etiology are arteriosclerosis and syphilis. Either condition may be the cause of aneurysms of the thoracic aorta, the comparative incidence varying with the rate of venereal infection. Only arteriosclerosis appears important as a cause of aneurysms of the abdominal aorta. Arteriosclerosis is also the chief cause of peripheral arterial aneurysms, except for those which result from an infected embolus. Peripherally, arteriosclerotic aneurysms occur in frequency in about the following order: popliteal artery, femoral artery, carotid artery and the intraabdominal and intrathoracic branches of the aorta.

The chronic symptoms of aneurysm are principally those produced by compression of surrounding structures. The actual dilatation and fundamental disease process notably cause discomfort only in active syphilitic infection of the thoracic aorta. The symptoms of arterial insufficiency are usually minimal, although an aneurysm produces some restriction in blood flow in proportion to the disturbance in efficient lamellar flow which the widening causes.

The serious hazards of arteriosclerotic and syphilitic aneurysms are rupture and thrombosis. The marked tendency for these complications to occur provides a strong indication for the removal of the lesion whenever recognized.

The rupture of an abdominal aortic aneurysm is not confined to lesions of large size. The fact that small ones rupture with some frequency suggests that thinning out of the stretched vascular wall is not the sole factor in disruption. Actually, the thinning process is compensated for by the development of an intraluminal mural thrombus (*A*) which may be a quite tough and rubbery mass. Inasmuch as this mural thrombus forms in such a way as to enclose the flow of blood through the remaining lumen in more or less the direct route through the lesion, it is apt to be less prominent in the region of the vertebral column than it is anteriorly, where the major volume of the aneurysm lies.

This comparative thinness of the mural clot in the region of the spine, together with the thinning which develops in the aneurysmal wall due to compression against the bony spine, are factors which are responsible for the location of the commonest point of rupture (*B*). This is posterior or dorsal, adjacent to the vertebral bodies, and usually the direction taken by the blood escaping from the aneurysm is to the left. Rupture is accompanied by prominent abdominal and back pain, signs of blood loss and development of a pulsating hematoma in the left flank.

Thinning of the anterior wall of the aneurysm (*C*) sometimes occurs and leads to rupture in that direction. (*D*). The resulting hematoma may remain confined for some time between the layers of the mesentery. Clinically, the aneurysm is found to have enlarged and abdominal pain is more prominent than back pain.

Arteriosclerotic aneurysm can also rupture into the inferior vena cava (*E* and *F*), just as the syphilitic variety in the chest can rupture into the superior vena cava. An explanation of this direction of rupture is occasionally seen in resection of a nonruptured aneurysm: the vena cava and aorta are densely adherent and the walls of both are quite thin in the area of contact. The disastrous acute heart failure that might be expected to follow this catastrophe is limited by the fact that the vena cava in the area of rupture is compressed to some extent by the arterial lesion.

Rupture of an aneurysm into the gastrointestinal tract may also be less spectacular than might be predicted. The intermittency of bleeding which can mark this event is due in part to compression of the loop of bowel involved and in part to plugging of the rupture site by a shift in the mural thrombus within the aneurysm.

PLATE 48

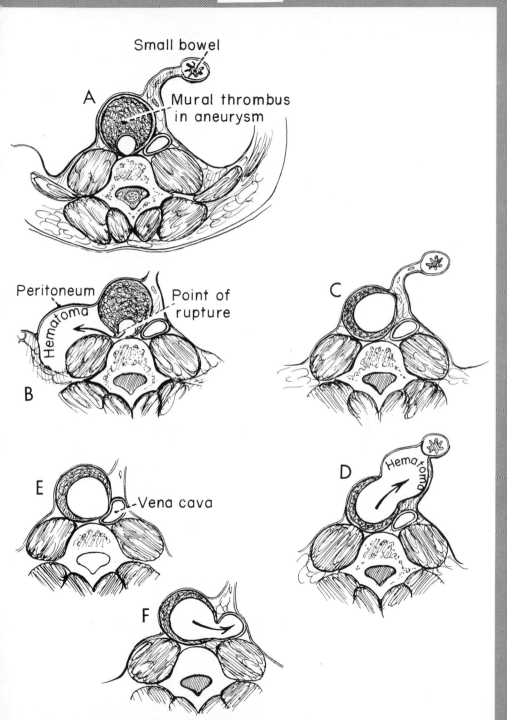

A — Small bowel — Mural thrombus in aneurysm

B — Peritoneum — Hematoma — Point of rupture

C

D — Hematoma

E — Vena cava

F

Resection and graft replacement of arteriosclerotic aneurysms of the abdominal aorta in the absence of complicating factors is accompanied by a very low mortality. The factors which increase mortality progressively, when present singly or in combination, are: coronary artery disease, marked obesity, disturbances in renal or pulmonary function, obstructive arterial disease in the legs and very advanced age. The single greatest cause of postoperative mortality in elective operations is myocardial infarction. However, the most important factor which adversely influences the outcome of operation is acute rupture. The strong tendency of aneurysms to rupture results in a decision to remove the aneurysm in most cases, even though factors increasing operative risk may be present.

Abdominal aneurysm resection is done through a full-length paramedian incision (*A*). After placement of a large self-retaining retractor, the bowel is retracted and carefully packed above and to the right of the incision on the abdominal wall. The posterior peritoneum is then opened between the root of the small bowel mesentery and the inferior mesenteric vein. Incision through the ligament of Treitz and mobilization of the last portion of the duodenum enhance exposure of the aneurysm neck.

The neck of the aneurysm is then mobilized just distal to the renal artery and below the left renal vein. The inferior mesenteric artery is ligated close to its origin to prevent injury to the collaterals in the mesentery. Finally, the iliac arteries are encircled below and prepared for clamping. The aneurysm is thus prepared for cross-clamping at the neck (*B*). While the aorta is cross-clamped, 20 mg. of heparin, diluted to 20 cc. with saline, is injected into the aneurysm. The aorta is then released for three or four beats and again cross-clamped below the renal arteries. Similarly, the iliac vessels are clamped with noncrushing vascular forceps. The anterior aspect of the aneurysm is longitudinally incised (*C*), and the laminated thrombus removed from the interior (*D*). Occasionally the aorta is not circumferentially divided if the posterior vessel wall is thin or is densely adherent. Occasionally the aortic bifurcation will be near normal, permitting its preservation and the eventual placement of a tube graft instead of a bifurcation graft.

[Resection and graft in abdominal aneurysm *continued on page 152.*]

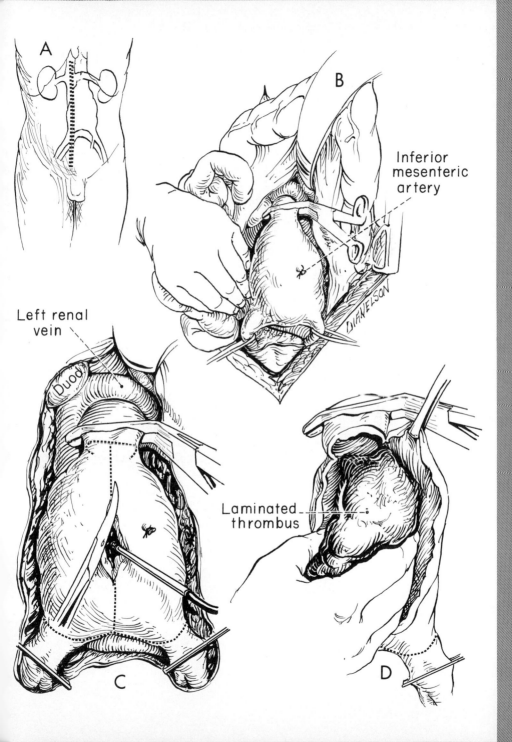

PLATE 49

A

B

Inferior
mesenteric
artery

DICKELSON

Left renal
vein

Duod

Laminated
thrombus

C

D

The aneurysm has been mobilized just sufficiently to permit isolation and control of the aorta and iliac vessels above and below the lesion as well as access to the anterior aspect of the aneurysm to permit its incision. No attempt is made to expose the posterior wall of the aneurysm or to control the lumbar branches. Efforts to mobilize the aneurysm further or to separate it from the cava are unnecessary and are apt to result in blood loss from venous injury.

After the laminated thrombus has been removed, the loosely adherent intima is separated from the outer fibrous wall of the aneurysm and peeled away where it is conveniently removed (*E*). Attention is then directed to any lumbar arteries which are bleeding and these are suture ligated (*F*). The bifurcation graft, which has been preclotted and trimmed to proper size, is then anastomosed end-to-end to the aorta. *G*, *H* and *I* illustrate the suturing techniques. The 000 Dacron sutures are usually begun at the posterior midline and each suture then placed around 50 per cent of the circumference to meet in the midline anteriorly. Occasionally, sutures at opposite corners may be preferable. A 2–3 mm. bite of the graft is taken and a 6–10 mm. bite used on the aortic side. Where possible, the graft is placed inside the aortic lip.

Care must be taken in forming the anastomosis to ensure that the suture is pulled up at right angles to the aorta to prevent cutting of the frequently fragile wall. Each suture must be individually tightened. A good method is to pull on the suture while placing reverse tension on the aorta at the point of suture emergence with a needle holder. Meticulous technique results in a negligible incidence of suture line leaks.

[Resection and graft in abdominal aneurysm *continued on page 154.*]

PLATE 49

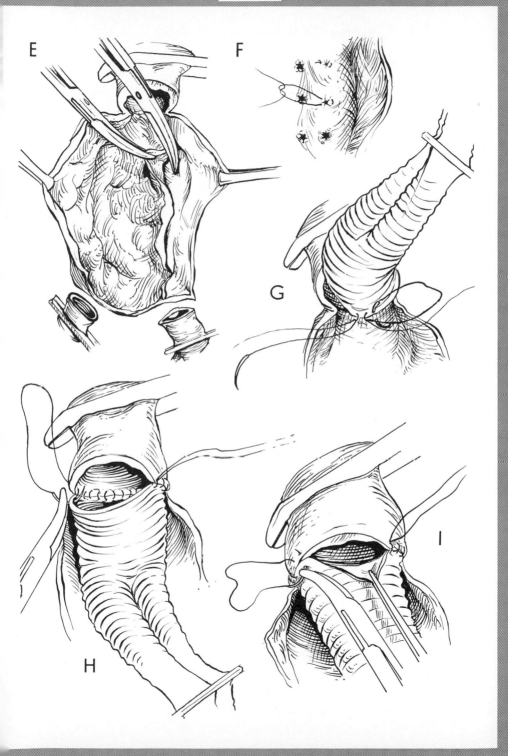

E

F

G

H

I

After the aortic anastomosis has been completed, one distal limb of the graft is then anastomosed. The anastomosis is most often made end-to-end to the common iliac artery but occasionally, either because of aneurysmal change in the common iliac or because of occlusive disease in this artery, it must be constructed end to side to the external iliac or even to the common femoral vessel. When an end-to-side distal anastomosis is used, the cut end of the common iliac artery must be closed with extreme care.

A 0000 Dacron suture is most often used for the distal anastomosis. Commonly, two sutures are started at the posterior midline and then each suture is applied over half the circumference to meet at the midline anteriorly. The graft is carefully tucked inside a cuff of distal artery when possible.

After one limb of the graft has been anastomosed, flow is permitted to that side by a careful sequence of clamp release. Initially, clamps are released in the iliac system to permit back bleeding from these vessels and hence to let blood exit from the yet unanastomosed graft limb. In the second maneuver the anastomosed limb of the graft is clamped and blood is briefly flushed through the aorta and out the unattached limb. Third, the free limb of the graft is cross-clamped and flow permitted from the aorta through the distal anastomosis and into the internal iliac artery (*J*). Finally, after blood has been washed through these channels, the external iliac artery is released.

Anastomosis of the other limb of the graft is carried out in a similar manner. The initial flow is then directed into the internal iliac channel. It is important that all clamps be released gradually to avoid abrupt changes in peripheral resistance and to avoid blood loss through the graft suture lines before fibrin and clot have had a chance to secure hemostasis.

With the functioning graft in place (*K*), the remnant of the aneurysm wall posteriorly is trimmed of its excess so that just enough remains to be sutured about the functioning prosthesis. The aneurysmal remnant is then carefully sutured over the graft (*L*) in such a way as to cover it, with particular attention given to the upper end where there is a need to interpose a barrier between the proximal anastomosis and the duodenum. Finally, the retroperitoneal tissues are closed over the aortic reconstruction with running sutures of catgut (*M*).

PLATE 49

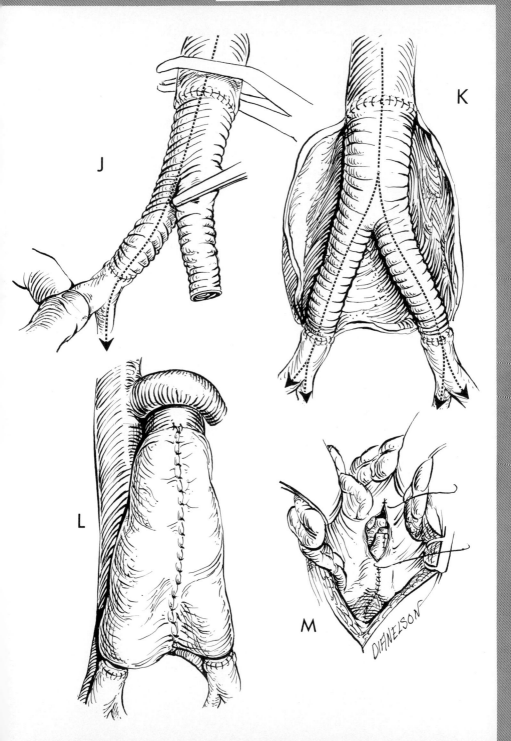

Aneurysms of the popliteal artery are the most common of the peripheral aneurysms. Almost all are caused by arteriosclerosis, with an occasional one being due to trauma or infection. They occur almost exclusively in males, are bilateral in 50 per cent of patients and in about 20 per cent there is an associated abdominal aortic aneurysm. Complications of these aneurysms are of four types. Most often popliteal aneurysms thrombose, with abrupt distal ischemia. Acute thrombosis results in a high incidence of limb loss through gangrene. The other consequences of popliteal aneurysms are rupture, pressure phenomena on the adjacent nerves and veins in the popliteal space and, finally, the production of small peripheral emboli. This fourth complication perhaps is due to the constant trauma to which the aneurysm is subjected due to knee action.

Resection is done under a general anesthesia with the patient positioned as shown in *A*. A Z-shaped incision is made to avoid a bowstring scar across the popliteal space. The popliteal artery is isolated at the upper end of the aneurysm, separating it from the adjacent popliteal vein (*B*). After distal heparinization the isolated popliteal arterial bifurcation is cross-clamped (*C*) and the aneurysm removed. Reconstruction of the popliteal artery is then done, usually with an autogenous saphenous vein graft. If a vein graft is not available then an 8 mm.-diameter prosthetic graft is used. Anastomoses are done in end-to-end fashion (*D*) with fine synthetic suture. The graft is shown in place in *E*.

PLATE 50

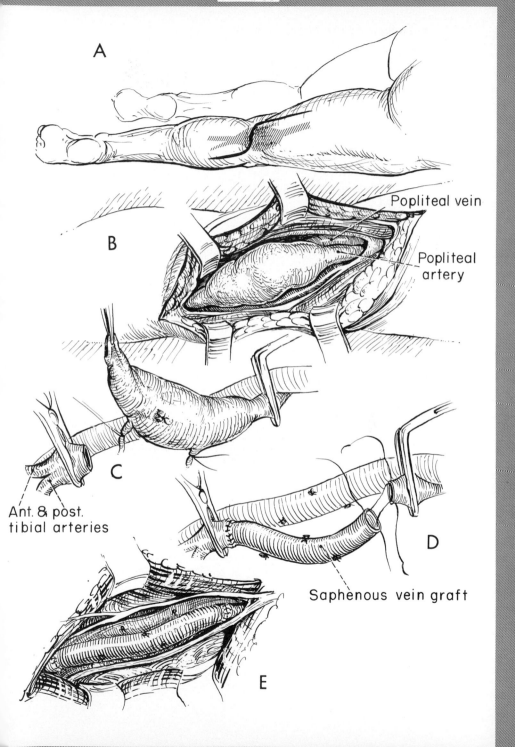

A

B

Popliteal vein

Popliteal artery

C

Ant. & post. tibial arteries

D

Saphenous vein graft

E

Saccular Aneurysm

A saccular aneurysm of the thoracic aorta develops because of the lack of elasticity in a patch of scar tissue in the wall of the aorta, the scar tissue resulting from healing of an area of aortitis, almost exclusively of the syphilitic type. These aneurysms usually have a pouchlike appearance, with a relatively narrow neck constituting the orifice between the aorta and the aneurysmal sac. This type of lesion has been seen at all levels of the thoracic aorta. Aortography is essential, not only to determine that the aneurysm is saccular rather than fusiform but also to locate the actual part of the arch involved.

LATERAL ANEURYSMECTOMY. — The saccular aneurysms that have a small neck involving less than one-half the circumference of the aorta are amenable to tangential excision and aortorrhaphy. In *A*, a saccular aneurysm arises from the anterior surface of the ascending limb of the aortic arch. A transverse thoracotomy is used to expose the root of the aorta, the mass of the aneurysm and the superior and inferior venae cavae for control with tapes. Undoubtedly a sternotomy is an alternative approach to this lesion. The wall of the aneurysm will be found adherent to the aorta for some distance from the orificial opening. This gives the aneurysm the appearance of having a much broader base than it actually has. Dissection in this area, carried along close to the wall of the normal aorta, serves progressively to narrow the amount of base of the aneurysm which must later be occluded with a clamp.

When dissection between the aneurysm and the aorta has been carried to its maximum extent, the aneurysm is held up and, with the superior and inferior venae cavae occluded for a moment or two, a long vascular forceps is applied. The venae cavae are released and transection of the base of the aneurysm is begun (*B*). As the aneurysm is cut from the aorta, interrupted sutures are placed, progressively closing the wall of the aorta. These interrupted sutures are reinforced (*C*) by a continuous over-and-over suture after the aneurysm is removed.

[Repair of thoracic aortic aneurysm using temporary by-pass *on page 160.*]

PLATE 51

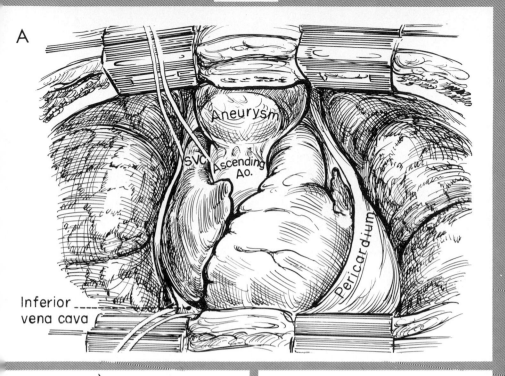

A

Aneurysm

SVC Ascending
Ao.

Pericardium

Inferior
vena cava

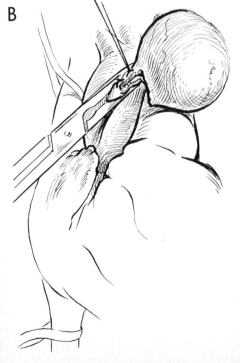

B

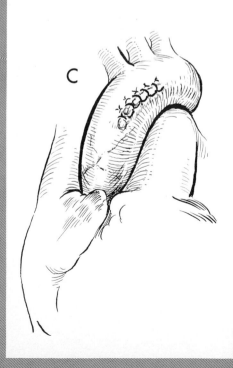

C

REPAIR USING TEMPORARY BY-PASS GRAFT.—In most instances the neck of the lesion is not well defined or involves more than 50 per cent of the circumference of the aorta. Under these circumstances, a temporary by-pass shunt between the proximal and distal aorta, total cardiopulmonary by-pass or femoral vein to femoral artery by-pass may be utilized to permit isolation of the aneurysm from the rest of the circulatory system. After excision of the aneurysm, if the resulting defect is large, a patch graft of Teflon or Dacron can be used to reconstruct the aorta.

In *A*, a tube graft is extended from the ascending to the descending aorta. This permits isolation of the segment of the ascending aorta from which the saccular aneurysm originated (*B*). However, a good portion of the proximal ascending aorta must be of normal size and quality to permit the insertion of a temporary by-pass graft. *B* and *C* illustrate primary suturing of the orifice to the aneurysm, using longitudinal closure. In *D*, because of the width of the defect and the fear of constriction of the aorta with a simple closure, an elliptic patch of Teflon has been used to reconstruct the ascending aorta. Removal of the temporary graft and suture closure of the anastomotic sites terminate the procedure.

PLATE 52

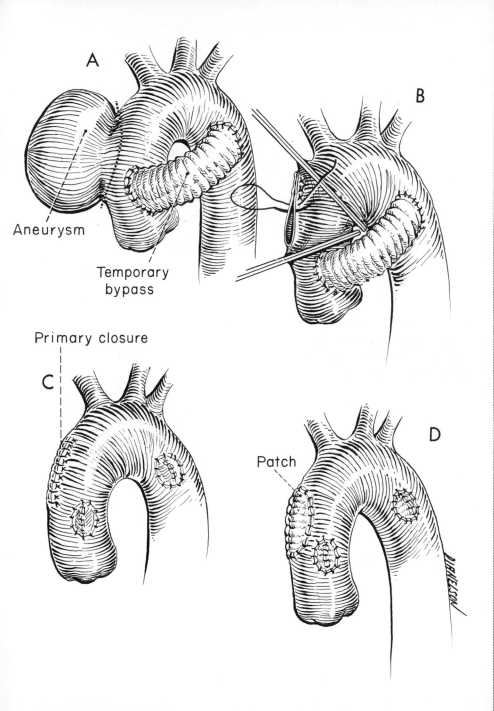

A

Aneurysm

Temporary
bypass

Primary closure

C

B

D

Patch

Fusiform Aneurysm

In resecting these aneurysms the important considerations stem from the necessity for temporary interruption of aortic flow through the segment to be resected. Important consequences of aortic occlusion are substantial increase in peripheral vascular resistance which may lead to left heart failure and possible ischemic damage to the vital structures distally, such as the spinal cord and the abdominal viscera. To overcome these problems, several methods have been used. One includes the use of hypothermia to protect sensitive structures from the effect of anoxia during the period of occlusion and the use of potent vasodilator drugs to diminish the degree of acute cardiac strain during the period of pronounced rise in peripheral resistance.

The second method consists of the use of a temporary by-pass shunt. This has been accomplished either by interposing a catheter between the subclavian and the left femoral arteries or by using a temporary by-pass graft sutured end-to-side to the aorta proximal and distal to the involved segment.

Because of the disadvantages of hypothermia and the limitations of the temporary by-pass shunts, controlled extracorporeal circulation has achieved widespread application. This may be accomplished by two different techniques. In the first technique, oxygenated blood is removed from the left atrium and pumped into the femoral artery (*A*). In the second technique, partial cardiopulmonary by-pass is achieved by cannulating the left common femoral artery and vein (*B*). The rate of flow is determined by the pressure proximal to the occluded aortic segment as measured preferably directly via catheter in the right ulnar artery. Systemic heparinization is necessary immediately prior to cannulation when left atriofemoral or venoarterial by-pass is employed. After the completion of the procedure, protamine sulfate is administered intravenously to neutralize the heparin.

If the aneurysm is well localized to the midportion of the descending aorta and the aorta is normal both proximally and distally, a sutured-in by-pass graft used as a temporary shunt is a satisfactory method of maintaining flow to the distal aorta while the aneurysm is resected and a graft placed (*C* and *D*).

[Resection and graft with cardiopulmonary by-pass *on page 164.*]

PLATE 53

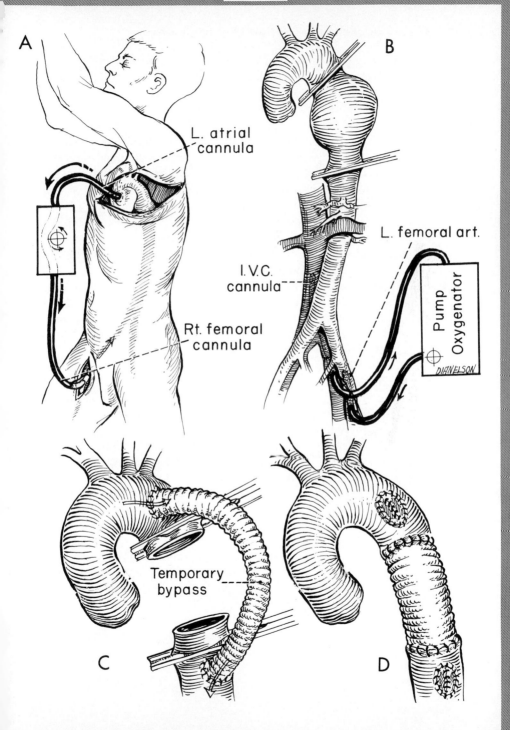

A

L. atrial
cannula

I.V.C.
cannula

Rt. femoral
cannula

B

L. femoral art.

Pump
Oxygenator

DIANELSON

Temporary
bypass

C

D

Fusiform aneurysms involve the entire circumference of the aorta; consequently, extirpational therapy requires resection of the diseased segment and a graft replacement. The preparation necessary to perform this procedure varies with the location of the lesion.

For the descending aorta, a generous left periscapular thoracotomy with the removal of the entire fifth rib provides adequate exposure. The lung, which is usually adherent to the pleura over the aneurysm, is separated by sharp dissection and retracted forward. The pleura over the lesion is incised longitudinally (*A*), the incision extending up along the subclavian artery. The vagus nerve is isolated and retracted medially. The recurrent laryngeal branch of the vagus is protected as the ligamentum arteriosum is being dissected. Ligation and division of the ligament early in the operation improves the mobility of the upper end of the aneurysm.

As much dissection as is possible of the aneurysm and of the aorta above and below it is done before by-pass of one of the types described on page 160 is indicated. However, some of the left intercostal arteries and usually most of those on the right side may not be ligated until the aneurysm has been transected above and below (*B*). Its greater mobility makes these vessels more readily accessible. Preparations are then made for the by-pass. Constant monitoring of the blood pressure proximal to the clamp determines the amount of blood that can safely be removed from the left atrium or femoral vein to be pumped into the femoral artery.

The aneurysm is excised between the clamps and a crimped, woven Dacron graft is inserted to reconstruct the descending aorta. The proximal anastomosis (*C*) is quickly done because the graft can be elevated to expose the posterior suture line. The posterior aspect of the distal suture line (*D*) is placed through the apposed lumens from in front. Just before completion of this anastomosis, the distal clamp is released briefly to force air from the graft. The anastomosis is then finished and the distal clamp is removed first to minimize the force which will come to bear on the suture lines.

PLATE 54

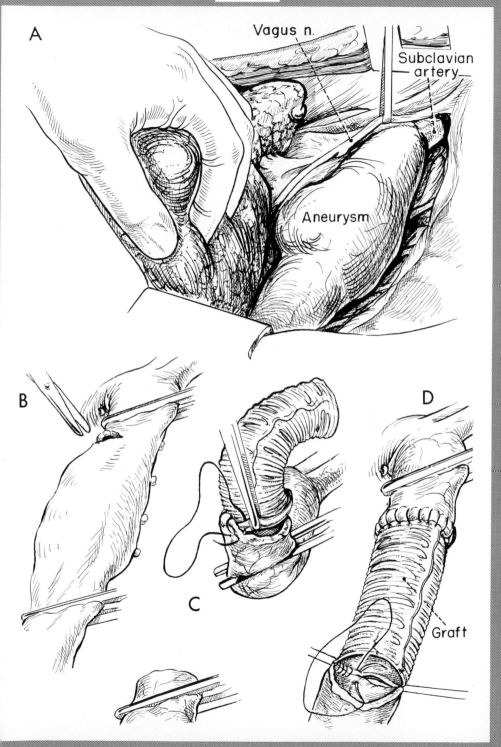

A

Vagus n.

Subclavian artery

Aneurysm

B

C

D

Graft

This type of lesion demands the use of a temporary total cardiopulmonary by-pass. A median sternotomy provides excellent exposure to the heart and the aneurysm. The method of cannulation for extracorporeal circulation is shown in *A*. The venous return into the oxygenator is by gravity via cannulas inserted into the superior and inferior venae cavae. Independent pumps are used for systemic and coronary perfusion. A left ventricular catheter attached to suction provides a dry field; it is used to prevent left ventricular distention and to aid in removing air from the left heart chambers after completion of the procedure.

With the patient on total by-pass, the ascending aorta is clamped distal to the aneurysm. Transection of the aorta superior to the aortic valve permits cannulation of the coronary arteries and restoration of myocardial perfusion. Dissection of the aneurysm from the surrounding structures, particularly the pulmonary artery, requires extra care and some is left behind if damage to these structures seems inevitable. In *B*, the aneurysm has been excised and the proximal anastomosis is begun. The proximal anastomosis is left incomplete to maintain coronary perfusion while the distal anastomosis is performed (*C*). Removal of the coronary catheters and completion of the proximal anastomosis permit release of the aortic clamp. Then, in the presence of satisfactory cardiac contractions, the pump-oxygenator can be discontinued (*D*).

PLATE 55

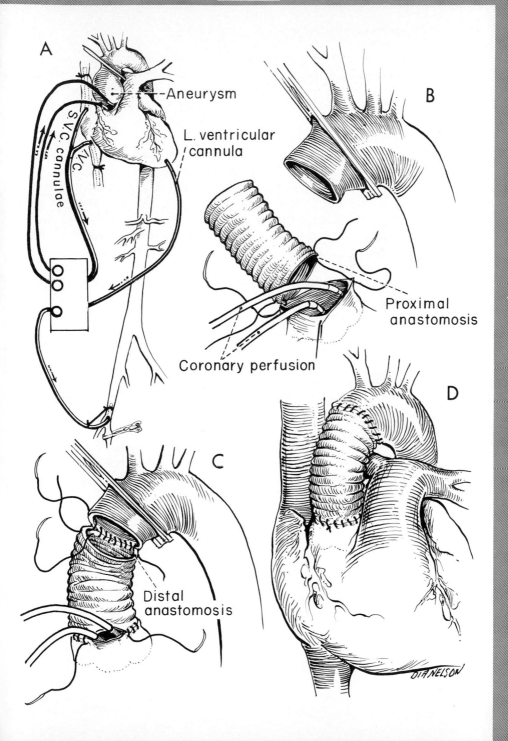

A

Aneurysm

S.V.C. cannula

I.V.C.

L. ventricular cannula

B

Proximal anastomosis

Coronary perfusion

C

Distal anastomosis

D

DIA NELSON

In certain patients with aortic root aneurysm, the aortic valve is incompetent and its correction becomes an essential part of the procedure. If the insufficiency is a result of dilatation of the valve ring, the procedure of choice is prosthetic replacement of the valve before the ascending aorta is reconstructed.

The commonest cause of aortic root aneurysm involving the sinuses of Valsalva is cystic medial necrosis, with or without other stigmas of Marfan's malformation. Under these circumstances the proximal aorta is extremely thin and friable. The method of cannulation is identical to the technique described for resection of an ascending aortic aneurysm (Plate 55).

A shows a typical aortic root aneurysm extending down to the valve. Annular dilatation, lack of valve support and intimal dissection extending to the commissures individually or in combination have been responsible for valvular regurgitation. In most instances, regardless of the mechanism of aortic insufficiency, valve replacement using a prosthetic valve is necessary to restore normal hemodynamics. In *B* the aneurysm has been excised, and in *C* a cage-ball valve prosthesis is being sutured to the aortic annulus. After insertion of the prosthetic valve, a tube graft is used to reconstruct the ascending aorta (*D* and *E*). Again, most of the proximal anastomosis is done first since at this time the exposure is optimal and a secure suture line can be achieved.

PLATE 56

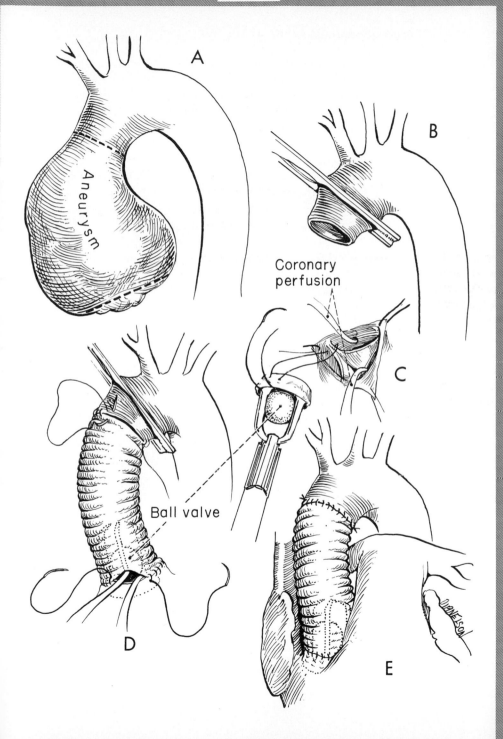

A

Aneurysm

B

Coronary
perfusion

C

Ball valve

D

E

Fusiform aneurysm involving the distal descending and upper abdominal aorta presents a surgical challenge primarily because of the involvement of the major branches to the abdominal organs — the celiac, superior mesenteric and renal arteries. Adequate exposure is achieved through a left thoracoabdominal incision extending from the midaxillary line obliquely across the costal margin and down as a longitudinal abdominal incision (*A*). The chest is entered through the sixth or seventh intercostal space. The left pleural and peritoneal cavities are entered and the diaphragm is incised radially to the aortic hiatus.

The abdominal organs are then mobilized to the right. This maneuver exposes the entire aorta and the aneurysm. The aorta above and below the aneurysm and the visceral branches are carefully dissected and encircled with cord tapes (*B*). A crimped, woven Dacron tube of appropriate size is then anastomosed end-to-side to the aorta proximal and distal to the involved segment, thus by-passing the aneurysm (*C*). Four Dacron tubes of smaller caliber, measuring approximately 6 – 10 mm. in diameter, are attached end-to-side to the original graft to be used to restore circulation to the celiac, superior mesenteric and renal arteries.

In positioning these side branches care should be taken to avoid subsequent malrotation or kinking of the grafts. The sequence of restoration of vascular continuity to the major abdominal branches is not important, since these vessels are reconstructed individually and at no time is more than one artery deprived of its circulation. Not infrequently one or more visceral branches may be partially or completely occluded proximally. If, for instance, the superior mesenteric artery is completely occluded at its origin, either because of laminated clots within the aneurysm or because of a chronic atherosclerotic process involving the initial portion of the artery itself, one has the choice of leaving the vessel obstructed or, if feasible, of undertaking the highly desirable restoration of normal circulation in the artery. Undoubtedly, in the presence of symptoms of arterial insufficiency to the intestinal tract, reconstruction of the occluded artery is essential.

[Resection and graft of thoracoabdominal aortic aneurysm *continued on page 172.*]

PLATE 57

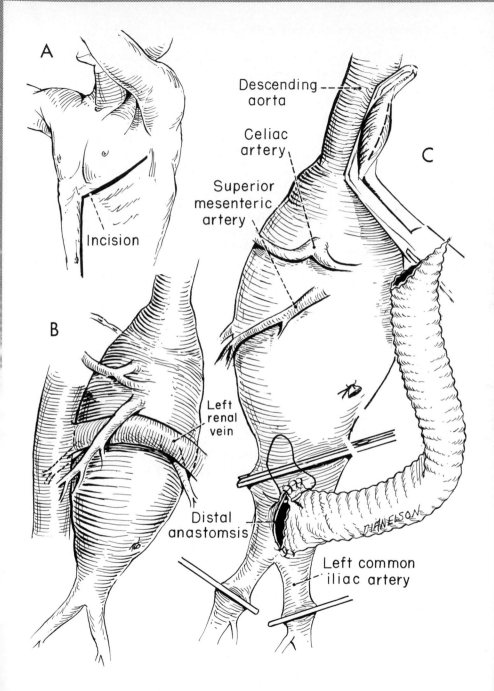

A

Incision

B

C

Descending aorta

Celiac artery

Superior mesenteric artery

Left renal vein

Distal anastomsis

Left common iliac artery

D.HNELSON

In *D*, the side grafts have been anastomosed to the distal divided ends of the celiac, superior mesenteric and left renal arteries. The partially occluding clamp has excluded a portion of the wall of the main graft in preparation for the fourth side graft, which will be used to restore flow to the right renal artery. In *E*, the right renal artery anastomosis is being performed while the flow has been established through other branches. *F* shows the completed reconstruction after resection of the aneurysm, including closure of the proximal divided end of the descending aorta and the almost completed closure of the divided end of the abdominal aorta.

With this technique the duration of ischemia to the abdominal viscera can be kept at a minimum. Heparinization has not been necessary during this operation. In certain patients temporary division of the left renal vein has been done to facilitate resection of the aneurysm.

PLATE 57

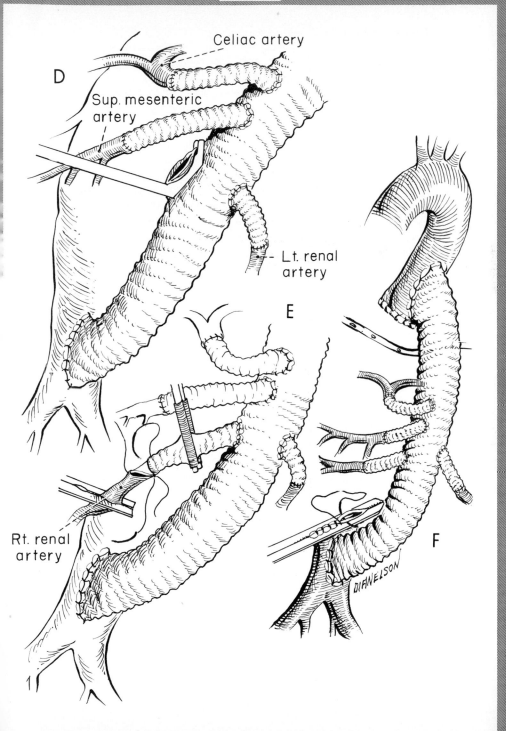

D

Celiac artery

Sup. mesenteric
artery

Lt. renal
artery

E

Rt. renal
artery

F

DIANELSON

1

Aneurysm of the aortic arch can be resected and the defect bridged either by the use of compound temporary by-passes or by the use of extracorporeal circulation. Selection of the procedure is primarily based on the extent of the involvement of the proximal aorta. The method of temporary aortic by-pass is applicable only when the proximal aorta is available for construction of a large end-to-side anastomosis with a prosthesis.

A bilateral transverse thoracotomy in the third interspace on the right and the fourth interspace on the left permits isolation of the ascending aorta, the arch branches and a small portion of the descending aorta. The possibilities in construction of the prosthesis to be used for by-pass are many. In *A*, the tube graft is shown being anastomosed distally to the descending aorta and proximally to the initial portion of the ascending aorta. In *B*, a bifurcation graft is anastomosed to the transverse tube graft with its limbs anastomosed to the sides of the innominate and left common carotid arteries. Circulation through the artery to which the appropriate limb of the graft is being sewn can be maintained by a temporary intraluminal shunt, which is removed immediately before the suture line is completed. Partially occluding clamps on the brachiocephalic vessels are not satisfactory for this purpose since the arteries are usually of small caliber.

In *B* the by-pass structures have been implanted and in *C* the aneurysm has been removed. At this time the ends of the involved arteries may be closed and a temporary by-pass left in place as the permanent replacement. If the arms of the by-passes are too long and the circulation through the various limbs is disproportionate, a carefully tailored prosthetic arch may be inserted (*D*). All the arch anastomoses are done while blood by-passes the region through the temporary shunts. The temporary prostheses are then removed and the points of lateral anastomoses closed.

PLATE 58

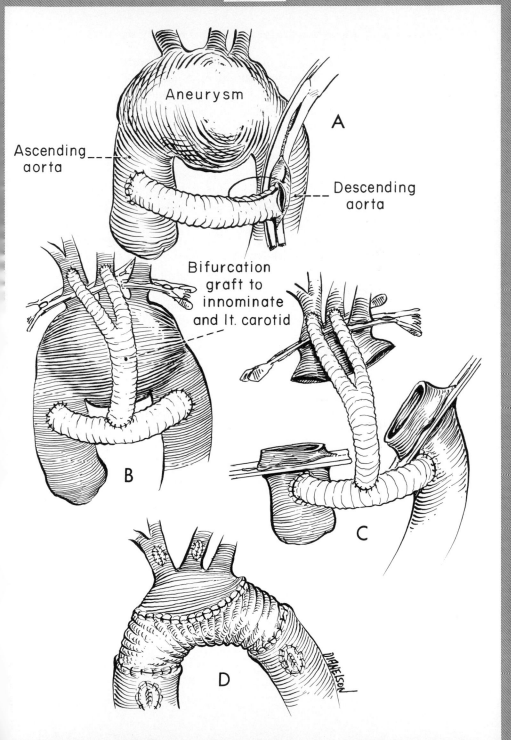

Aneurysm

Ascending aorta

Descending aorta

A

Bifurcation graft to innominate and lt. carotid

B

C

D

An aneurysm involving both the ascending aorta and the arch demands the use of extracorporeal circulation, using the pump-oxygenator plus various accessory arterial inflow leads. The need for and the number of cranial leads depend on whether the aneurysm involves the innominate or left carotid artery origin or both.

The pump connections for resection of an aneurysm which involves all the brachiocephalic branches are illustrated and diagramed in *A* and *B*. Venous blood is removed from the superior and inferior venae cavae, which are occluded with tapes. This blood is oxygenated and then pumped back through leads to the femoral artery, to each carotid artery and to the coronary arteries. Independent pumps for these arterial lines permit regulation and maintenance of desirable flow and pressure in each channel.

In this particular resection, with the patient in total by-pass, a clamp is placed on the descending aorta distal to the left subclavian artery, the carotids are cannulated and the brachiocephalic arteries are clamped at their origins. The aorta is then transected above the valve and the coronary arteries are cannulated for perfusion and maintenance of myocardial oxygenation. Cerebral perfusion is maintained through the two carotid and the right vertebral arteries. The resection of the aneurysm can be done very rapidly after completing these arrangements. A crimped Dacron tube graft is being utilized to reconstruct the aortic arch, as illustrated in *C*.

[Aortic arch resection using total cardiopulmonary by-pass *continued on page 178.*]

PLATE 59

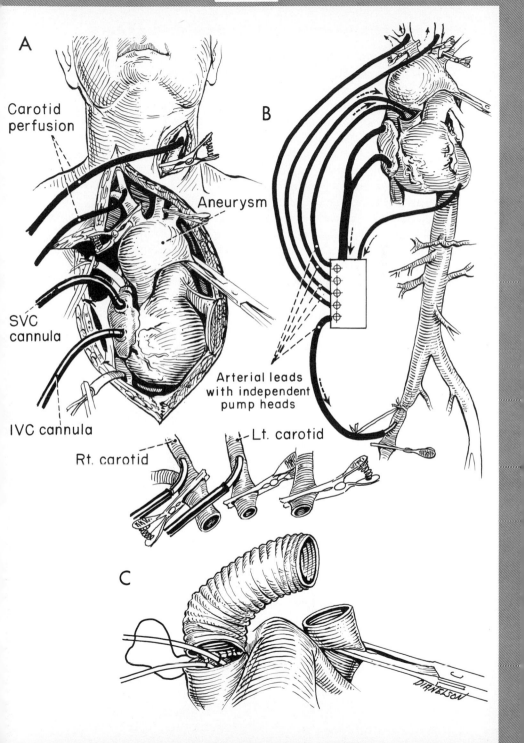

A

Carotid
perfusion

B

Aneurysm

SVC
cannula

IVC cannula

Arterial leads
with independent
pump heads

Lt. carotid

Rt. carotid

C

DANELSON

As shown in *D*, completion of the reconstruction of the main graft permits release of the clamp from the descending aorta, thereby restoring retrograde coronary perfusion. In *E*, the proximal divided ends of the three brachiocephalic arteries are directly anastomosed to the superior aspect of the graft. The temporary shunts have been removed from the carotids and the small arterotomies repaired. *F* illustrates brachiocephalic reconstruction using suitable side grafts sewn to the original prosthesis.

An extremely high operative mortality is associated with this operation, and among the causes of death irreversible cerebral damage is the most common and most challenging to prevent. Based on the metabolic requirements of the brain and the physical and physiologic cerebral blood flow, each cranial lead should receive at least 300–400 ml. of blood per minute. Contrast studies of the carotid and vertebral arteries before surgery will prove helpful in the proper management of cerebral circulation during cardiopulmonary by-pass. Restoration of circulation to all three brachiocephalic vessels assures maximum protection to the brain regardless of the preoperative state of the cerebral blood supply.

[Alternate method in aortic arch resection *on page 180.*]

PLATE 59

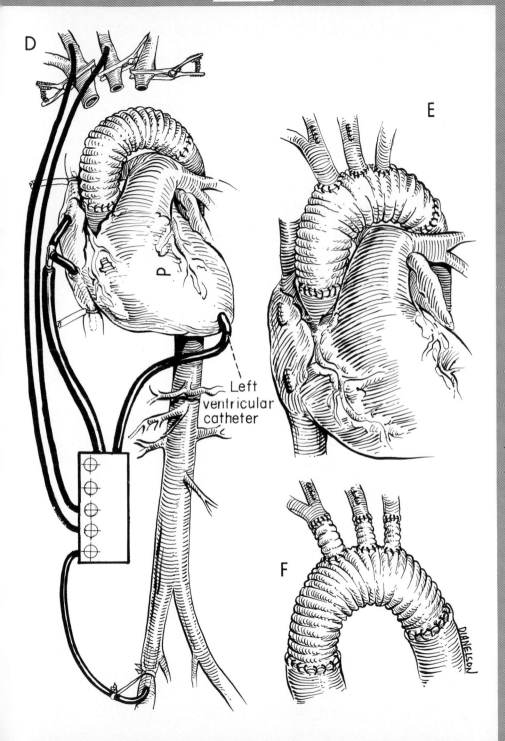

D

P

Left
ventricular
catheter

E

F

DJ NELSON

An alternative method of maintaining cerebral perfusion is illustrated in Plate 60. Preliminary preparations are similar to those for the previous technique. The patient is placed on total by-pass and the aneurysm is excluded by clamping the descending aorta and the cerebral vessels. The ascending aorta is transected superior to the coronary orifices at the site where the proximal anastomosis will be made. A tube graft of suitable size, with an opening in its superior aspect to correspond with the part of the wall of the aortic arch containing the orifices to the brachiocephalic arteries, is used (*A*). Two catheters connected to independent pumps are passed through the tube graft and its side opening and are extended from within the aneurysm into the innominate and left carotid arteries. These catheters are kept in place with Romel-type tourniquets around the base of each vessel. Arterial flow can then be established into the carotid arteries, and this, in addition, results in retrograde perfusion of the right vertebral branch. This technique of cannulation requires a brief interruption of cerebral blood flow, not exceeding a few minutes. If necessary, mild to moderate hypothermia can be used for added safety.

Anastomosis of the graft to the descending aorta and to the aortic cuff containing the brachiocephalic orifices (*B* and *C*) permits the removal of the carotid catheters, release of the descending aortic clamp and restoration of cerebral blood flow (*D*). The graft, of course, is clamped proximal to the origin of the innominate artery. Proximal anastomosis with removal of the coronary catheters (*E*) and restoration of effective cardiac contractions is followed by cessation of the pump-oxygenator.

PLATE 60

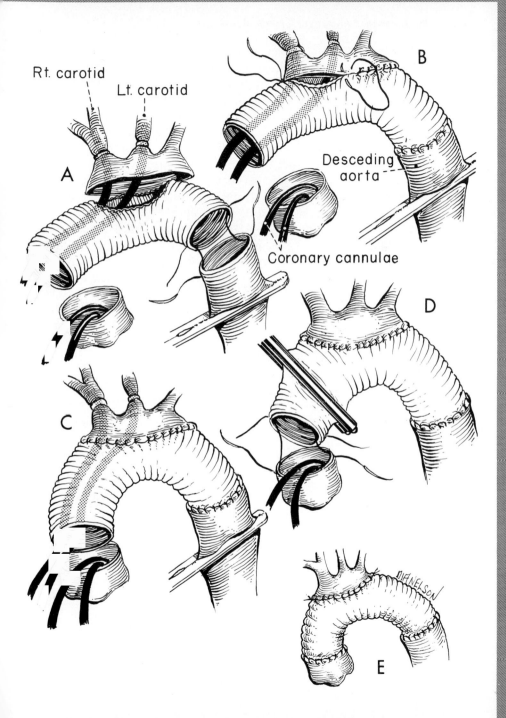

Rt. carotid   Lt. carotid

A

B

Desceding
aorta

Coronary cannulae

C

D

E

Two forms of aneurysm which are properly termed dissecting aneurysm characteristically appear at the upper descending thoracic aortic level and are amenable to resection using the same principles as those employed in arteriosclerotic aneurysms in this area. These lesions are (1) traumatic thoracic aneurysm, which is most frequently located in this position, and (2) the local dissecting aneurysm which develops when blood escapes out into the wall of the aorta through the edge of an arteriosclerotic plaque or ulcer. These forms of dissecting aneurysm remain localized longitudinally, whereas those which have as their pathogenesis a degenerative change in the media of the aorta often do not.

A shows the relation of the left fourth interspace thoracotomy incision to the lesion. In *B*, the isolation and resection of the aneurysm are indicated; the steps, including those in preparation for occlusion of the aorta, are the same as those illustrated in Plates 54 and 55.

The pathologic anatomy of the usual traumatic aneurysm is shown in *C* and *D*. The inner layers of media are usually torn transversely by the trauma, and an aneurysmal dilatation of the outer layers of the media and the adventitia occurs.

E and *F* indicate the origin of a localized dissecting aneurysm occurring in a severely arteriosclerotic aorta. Escape of blood into a layer between the coats of the vessel has been permitted by a tear in the inner layers at the site of fracture or ulceration of an atherosclerotic plaque.

Resection of the aneurysm is followed by replacement with a prosthetic tube (*G*).

PLATE 61

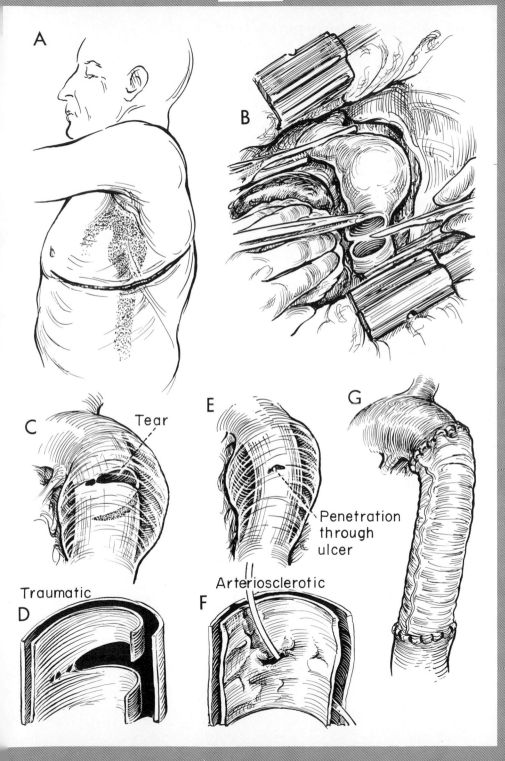

A

B

C Tear

E

G

Penetration through ulcer

Traumatic

D

Arteriosclerotic

F

An extremely bad prognosis accompanies the diagnosis of dissecting aneurysm either when it originates from a medial tear in the ascending aorta, or when it extends diffusely proximally and distally from a tear in the inner layers at the descending aortic level. The hazardous surgery which is undertaken in an attempt to save the patient is indicated because of the otherwise almost certainly fatal course of the disease. Two procedures are illustrated in Plates 62 and 63.

INTRALUMINAL DRAINAGE

Intraluminal drainage of the dissecting lumen is carried out through a generous left thoracotomy incision. Temporary by-pass from the left atrium to the femoral artery or partial cardiopulmonary by-pass using the common femoral artery and vein will be desirable. The usual structure of a dissected aorta is shown in *A*. The upper segment of the descending thoracic aorta is freed from surrounding structures and isolated between clamps. When it is transected, the double-barreled characteristic of the lesion is immediately apparent, and the distal end of the vessel is totally reconstructed by suture closure of the dissected lumen (*B*). Three-fourths to four-fifths of the circumference of the proximal cut end is similarly treated. The remaining segment of circumference is left open, and a portion of the inner cylinder is resected at this point to provide a window through which blood may flow from outer to inner lumen (*C*) after the vessel has been reanastomosed.

This procedure mimics a spontaneous re-entry of the dissected lumen. The technique has been generally superseded by procedures which attack the primary problem of the original tear. An example is illustrated in Plate 63.

PLATE 62

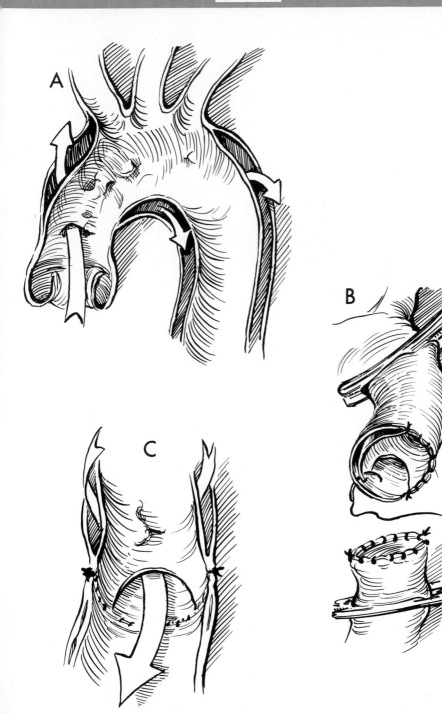

DIRECT REPAIR

Dissecting aneurysm arising immediately superior to the aortic valve may produce significant aortic regurgitation in addition to the other manifestations of distal dissection. Therefore, the surgical objectives should include repair of the aortic disruption, obliteration of the false lumen and restoration of valvular competence. To accomplish these, the surgical procedure may vary from primary repair of the defect to the replacement of both the valve and the ascending aorta. The technique of aortic valve replacement is illustrated in Plate 93. As to the replacement of the ascending aorta, the only modification from the technique illustrated in Plate 55 is that the divided ends of the aorta proximally and distally may be partially or completely double-barreled. In this case, the dissected layers are first approximated before the graft is inserted to replace the ascending aorta.

A shows a typical type I aortic dissection. As usual, the point of entry is immediately superior to the aortic valve. In *B*, the dissected layers are being approximated before primary end-to-end anastomosis (*C*) is carried out. Not infrequently the poor quality of the ascending aorta necessitates its resection (*D*) and the interposition of a tube graft (*E*) to restore aortic continuity.

This approximation on the proximal side stabilizes and supports the valve cusps which had been allowed to prolapse by the detachment of the intimal continuations of the commissures.

PLATE 63

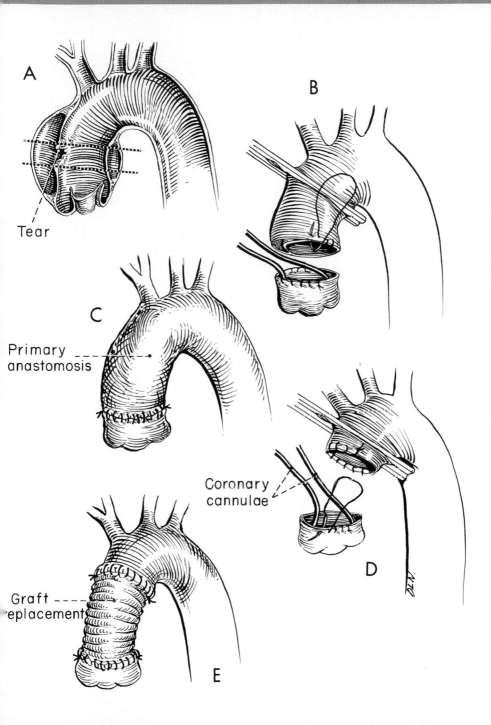

A

Tear

B

C

Primary
anastomosis

Coronary
cannulae

D

Graft
replacement

E

The Venous System

CHAPTER 10

General Considerations

THE MAJOR pathologic conditions affecting the venous system include compression from lesions of the surrounding tissues, thrombosis, inflammation, structural changes leading to dilatation and valvular incompetency, and trauma. An excellent example of a major vein which is effectively obstructed by lesions of the surrounding tissue is the superior vena cava. This vessel from its point of origin at the confluence of the two innominate veins down to the point of emptying into the right atrium is vulnerable to mediastinal neoplasm, arterial aneurysm and inflammations of the mediastinum. The scar tissue formation accompanying healing of mediastinal inflammation is surgically the most prominent cause of vena caval obstruction, so far as the surgery directly involves the vein. In conditions of compression of the superior vena cava by tumor or aneurysm, or similar compressions of the inferior vena cava and notably of the popliteal vein by aneurysm, the vein surgery is only an incident of the surgical management of the fundamental lesion.

Thrombosis of the lumen of a vein and inflammation of its wall are usually coincident processes, although one or the other may be a more outstanding feature. The importance of the intraluminal clot in vein thrombosis arises in part because it may become detached, with consequent pulmonary embolism, and in part because it represents an obstruction to blood flow. The phlebitic or inflammatory element is significant because it produces venous obstruction, causes destruction and inactivation of the valves and may extend from the vein wall to the surrounding lymphatics, thus increasing the degree of stasis of the tissues drained by the vein.

Varicose veins in the lower extremity represent the structural and functional disturbance produced by stretching of vein walls. When the cause is a primary weakness in the vein wall, hormonal relaxation of the muscularis of the vein secondary to pregnancy or an occupational stress, such as that in persons who stand a great deal, the varicose veins are termed "primary." "Secondary" varicose veins are those which develop when the subcutaneous venous system contributes to the general dilatation during the development of collateral venous channels in individuals whose major deep leg veins have been obstructed by some other process, predominantly thrombophlebitis. Trauma involving the major venous channels of a part has special importance, because it may potentiate the severity of an accompanying arterial injury or of itself may produce damaging acute venous insufficiency. Vein trauma is most apt to be serious when it accompanies a crushing injury of the part or when it occurs with a fracture, particularly one at the knee or elbow, which causes not only the vein injury but inactivates the collateral venous channels because of edema.

The facility with which arterial occlusions are repaired by thromboendarterectomy and graft procedures does not yet extend to repair of venous obstructions. An obstruction of the superior vena cava, the lesion which ought to respond most favorably to restorative surgery, remains difficult to manage. Despite the fact that the segment of involved vein is short and the flow produced by restoration is rapid and almost obligatory, restorations often fail.

The treatment of conditions associated under the term of thrombophlebitis is chiefly concerned with depression of the coagulation system by medical management. Surgery is used principally as an adjunct to prevent the occurrence of pulmonary embolism and, in the late stages of the disease, to help correct the sequelae of venous insufficiency. Removal of the intraluminal clot from the vein is sometimes useful if done very early in the acute stages of mildly inflammatory thrombophlebitis.

Uncomplicated primary varicose veins of the lower extremities produce few symptoms beyond aching and fatigue which occur after long periods of standing. The primary indication for treating these veins surgically is to prevent the complications of varicose veins. The common complications are a superficial phlebitis developing in the varicose channels and a seemingly increased liability to development of deep thrombophlebitis. Less frequently, the derangement of cutaneous venous drainage caused by primary varices in the lower part of the leg may be severe enough to produce such changes as eczema, fibrosis and finally ulceration.

Removal of varicose veins secondary to a deep thrombophlebitis is only a portion of the surgical therapy required in these patients. The stasis resulting from deep thrombophlebitis is much greater than that from primary varicose veins, because of the added elements of defective deep venous drainage and damage to the lymphatics at the time of the acute inflammation. Marked incompetence of the perforating veins in the lower leg also contributes to the stasis changes in the skin. The pigmentation, scarring, and ultimate breakdown of the skin characteristically are located along the medial aspect of the lower third of the leg where the disturbance from the perforating veins is greatest. These veins, which are communications between the deep and superficial venous systems of the leg, are usually four in number, are arranged longitudinally and in the state of health have valves that permit blood to flow only from the superficial to the deep systems. Phlebitis destroys the valves of these fascia-perforating veins and, thereafter, with the action of the calf musculature functioning as a venous pump, blood is ejected through the incompetent channels into the superficial channels. The result is an increase in the effect of venous stasis at the ankle. Treatment of such a damaged extremity must include, among other requirements, eradication of the incompetent perforating veins.

In the event that an ulcer is present, or if skin changes are so severe as to be irreversible, surgical treatment must in addition provide for the excision and skin graft replacement of the damaged tissue. Removal of tissue in the stasis area followed by skin grafting is not often necessary when the cause of the lesion is primary varicose veins without deep venous insufficiency. It is the more severe stasis, both venous and lymphatic, that causes the irreversible changes requiring excision and grafting.

The chronic stasis which follows deep thrombophlebitis can always be minimized and sometimes prevented by beginning management as the acute process subsides. Proper management prolongs the initial disability but in the end is timesaving. It consists of rigid prevention of edema by a gradual resumption of activity within whatever restrictions are necessary. Ambulation is begun only after all swelling of the acute attack has subsided. Then a period of walking is permitted each hour. This is gradually increased as each increment is demonstrated not to cause edema. Only after consolidation of the ambulatory periods has led to significant activity is external compression with elastic support started. The prevention of edema from the beginning provides the favorable environment necessary for formation of efficient collateral channels.

Surgical removal of varicose veins of the lower extremities, whether of primary or secondary type, requires painstaking thoroughness and accuracy to obtain satisfactory immediate results and to minimize recurrences. In most instances, both saphenous systems are involved and it is fundamental that the point of entrance of each into the deep circulation be exactly identified to avoid confusion in the presence of the frequent variations which are encountered. Ligation and division of the long saphenous vein at its junction with the common femoral vein and of the short saphenous at its junction with the popliteal is followed by removal of the vein in each instance. This is accompanied by direct excision of masses of varices, by additional stripping of any enlarged major tributaries of each saphenous channel and by exposure and interruption of perforating veins.

CHAPTER 11

Varicose Veins

Ligation and Stripping of Long Saphenous Vein

THE ENTIRE procedure is best done under general anesthesia, although the initial stage in the upper femoral triangle can
be carried out under local anesthesia (*A*). An obliquely transverse
incision paralleling Poupart's ligament is most frequently used
(*B*). In thin individuals, Poupart's ligament corresponds very closely
to the location of the inguinal crease, while obesity results in a
proportional downward displacement of the inguinal fold in relation
to the ligament. The incision extends from a point just lateral to the
palpable femoral artery pulse medially for a distance of 2 1/2 – 3 in.
It is developed through the superficial fat, exposing the superficial
femoral fascia, which is incised (*B*). Further dissection exposes the
superficial venous system, which is thoroughly dissected down to
the foramen ovale (*C*). Ligation and division of the tributaries of
the saphenous vein (*D*) are carried out as each is encountered. Absolute identification of the junction with the common femoral vein
requires some degree of isolation of the latter. When ligation of the
saphenous channel is properly done, the anterior wall of the vein
becomes flush with the ligated stump of the saphenous (*E*).

The stripper may be introduced from above downward (*F*), although in this direction its advancing tip sometimes engages the
superiorly oriented valve leaflets. Alternatively, it is passed from
below upward after the long saphenous vein has been exposed at
the level of the ankle. In either case, the upper end of the vein is
securely tied around the wire of the stripper so that traction upon it
will withdraw the vein (*G*).

[Ligation and stripping of long saphenous vein *continued on page 196*.]

PLATE 64

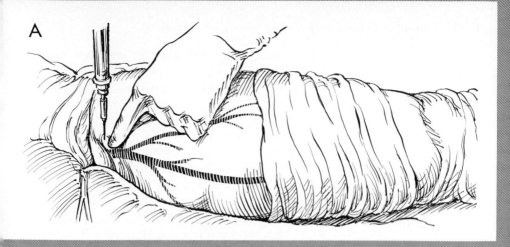

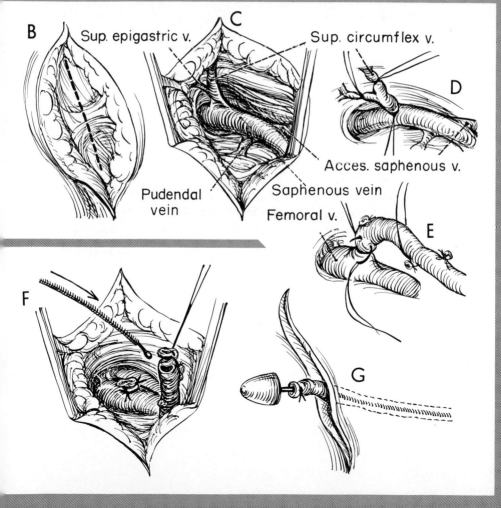

A

B

C Sup. epigastric v.

Sup. circumflex v.

D

Acces. saphenous v.

Pudendal
vein

Saphenous vein

Femoral v.

E

F

G

Withdrawal of the stripper with the vein may in actuality be done in either direction with the stripper in place (*H* and *I*). The points of entrance of previously noted large tributaries are exposed through additional incisions (*I*). One common location for such veins is on the medial aspect of the upper calf. Depending on their size, these veins either are simply ligated or are individually threaded with a stripper for secondary removal. As the vein is withdrawn, firm compression over much of its tract (*J*) will minimize bleeding under the skin. The blood that accumulates in the tract from which the vein has been removed may be expressed by a gentle milking action toward the skin incisions before they are closed.

The accessory saphenous vein in the thigh may be a very well-developed, though tortuous, channel requiring stripping. In addition, ligation and stripping of the lesser saphenous vein will be required in most cases.

PLATE 64

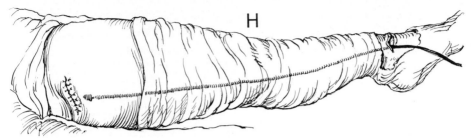

H

Stripper in long saphenous vein

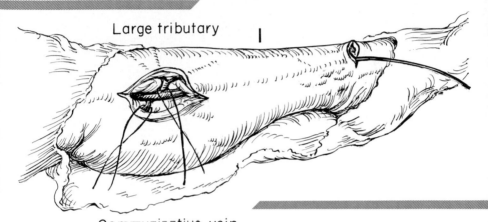

Large tributary

I

Communicative vein
to short saphenous

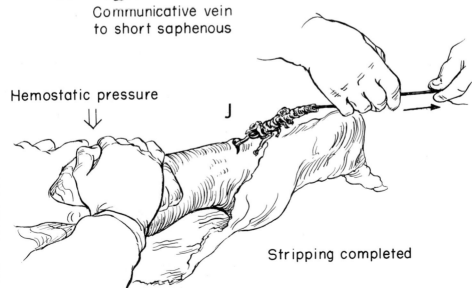

Hemostatic pressure

J

Stripping completed

The commonest cause of recurrence of varices of the long saphenous system is the incomplete interruption of the venous channels which enter the long saphenous vein at its point of connection to the common femoral vein. Variation in the positions of the various tributaries of the saphenous at this point are frequent. The major areas drained into the long saphenous vein are the superficial tissues of the pubis, the lower abdomen, the lateral iliac crest, the lateral surface of the upper thigh and the extensive drainage system entering the major channel itself from points on down the extremity. Four tributaries are ordinarily received by the long saphenous trunk in the region of the foramen ovale (*A*). These are the external pudendal vein, the superficial epigastric, the superficial circumflex iliac and the accessory saphenous veins. These are usually thought of as entering a major saphenous trunk, the ligation of which completely removes these veins from the influence of the incompetence of the saphenofemoral valve. Variations in the anatomy mislead the surgeon into leaving some of the tributaries in communication with the common femoral vein so that connections may be re-established later to portions of the saphenous bed below, causing recurrence.

The left superficial epigastric vein is illustrated (*A*) entering the common femoral vein above the major saphenofemoral junction. The distance between these two connections varies, but it may be great enough that the saphenous vein could be ligated leaving the superficial epigastric behind. Another variation is concerned with aberrant locations of the external pudendal artery. Normally (*B*) this artery traverses the lower edge of the foramen ovale in the deep fascia, lying, therefore, superficial to the common femoral vein and beneath all branches of the saphenous vein. This artery may occupy an anomalous position, crossing beneath the accessory saphenous vein and superficial to the saphenous itself (*C*), or it may lie superficial to all of the saphenous trunk except the superficial epigastric vein (*D*). In either instance, if the artery is used as a landmark for ligation, the surgeon will be in error. In the former instance he will ligate the accessory saphenous, leaving the major channel intact, while in the latter he will at best interrupt the major drainage from below, leaving the superficial epigastric vein for recurrence.

PLATE 65

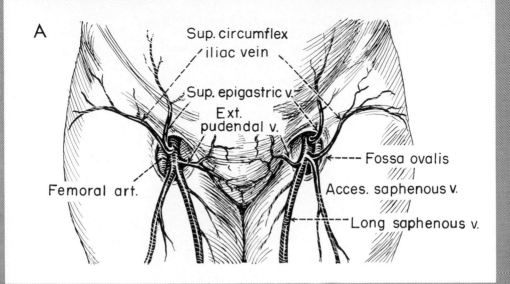

A

Sup. circumflex iliac vein

Sup. epigastric v.

Ext. pudendal v.

Femoral art.

Fossa ovalis

Acces. saphenous v.

Long saphenous v.

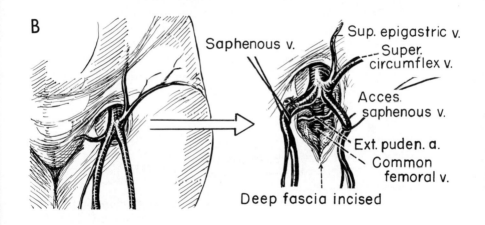

B

Saphenous v.

Sup. epigastric v.

Super. circumflex v.

Acces. saphenous v.

Ext. puden. a.

Common femoral v.

Deep fascia incised

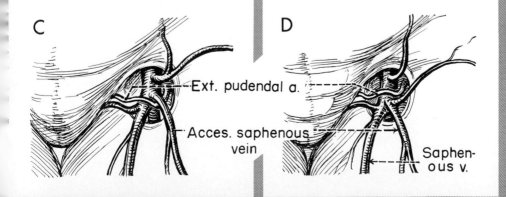

C

Ext. pudendal a.

Acces. saphenous vein

D

Ext. pudendal a.

Acces. saphenous

Saphenous v.

Removal of the short saphenous system by stripping is necessary for the complete eradication of varicose veins in most patients in whom removal of the long saphenous vein is indicated. For complete eradication of the short saphenous system, ligation of the vein near its point of entrance into the popliteal vein is necessary, care being taken that no tributary remains in communication with the popliteal. Exposure of this portion of the popliteal space in a patient who is undergoing ligation and stripping of both superficial venous systems bilaterally is particularly a problem in patients with very heavy legs. It can usually be done by internal rotation of the extremity with the knee flexed, as illustrated in *A*. However, if complicated masses of varices are present in the popliteal spaces, it may be desirable first to complete the long saphenous vein surgery and then to roll the patient entirely over onto an adjacent cart covered with a sterile drape in order to do the popliteal space surgery more conveniently.

A transverse incision is desirable in the popliteal space. This should be made a short distance distal to the major flexion crease. The vein lies lateral to the midline posteriorly and at this level is almost always beneath the sural fascia. When it is enlarged, it is not difficult to identify. It can be most quickly found if a stripper is passed from below upward before the popliteal incision is deepened through the fascia.

The short saphenous vein is exposed at the ankle through a longitudinal incision midway between the posterior border of the lateral malleolus and the achilles tendon. The vein, isolated at this point, is incised and a flexible stripper passed through the opening upward to the popliteal space (*B*).

The short saphenous vein, now positively identified in the popliteal space, is followed upward to visualize the popliteal vein and then ligated proximal to all tributaries. The tributaries are doubly ligated and divided as shown in *C*. Then the saphenous vein itself is incised, the stripping wire brought out through the end, attached to a suitably sized head and withdrawn by traction from below (*D*). Blood is expressed gently from the subfascial and subcutaneous tracts of the vein and the incisions closed.

PLATE 66

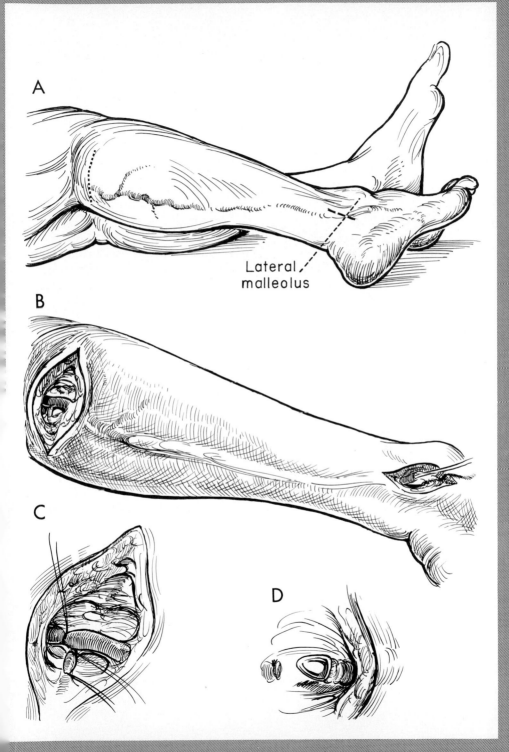

A

Lateral
malleolus

B

C

D

CHAPTER 12

Stasis Disease

Excision of Stasis Ulcer and Skin Graft

THE MAJOR soft-tissue changes which result from long-standing vein disease are atrophy and pigmentation of the skin; fibrosis; calcification of the subcutaneous tissue, and liquefaction with some saponification of the subcutaneous fat. The typical center of involvement is above the medial malleolus. The frequency with which these changes occur is far greater in extremities in which the deep venous system is insufficient than in those involved only by primary varicose veins. The localization of the process depends in either instance on the fact that this area is most affected by a combination of incompetence of the superficial venous system and incompetence of the perforating communications between the deep and superficial venous systems, these being most concentrated in this area.

The requirement in surgical treatment is the complete removal and ligation of incompetent superficial veins and the perforating veins, plus the removal of those tissues in the area which have undergone irreversible change. Excision of the stasis area is followed by application of a free split-thickness skin graft.

It is not always necessary to wait for complete healing of ulcers, but bacteriologic control prior to surgery is important. The leg is thoroughly prepared (A). The long saphenous system is subjected to proximal ligation. The stripper is placed in the vein (Plate 64) before the area of ulceration is attacked. Excision is carried out peripheral to the stasis area, the incision being in flexible tissue. During dissection beneath the deep fascia, perforating branches are encountered and ligated (B).

[Stasis ulcer excision and skin graft *continued on page 204*.]

PLATE 67

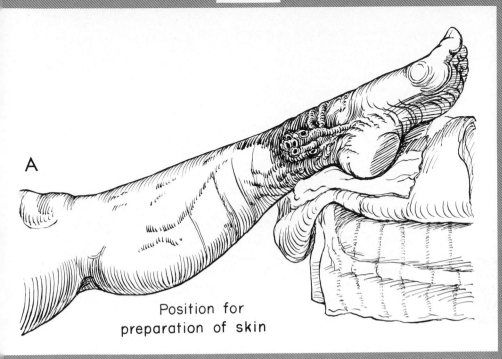

A

Position for
preparation of skin

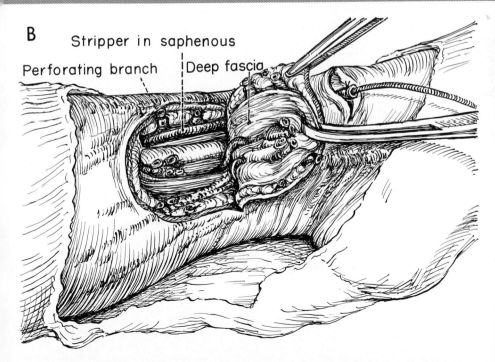

B

Stripper in saphenous

Perforating branch   Deep fascia

The split-thickness skin graft shown in *C* has been taken from the skin of the same thigh before the open or recently healed ulcer area is handled. This is done to minimize contamination of the donor site. For the same reason, the ligation of the saphenous vein and the introduction of the stripper are done early in the procedure. The major varicose tributaries to the saphenous vein in thigh and upper calf have been ligated. The incision in the groin has been closed and one incision in the upper medial calf has been sutured.

At this stage in the operation (*D*), the vein is removed by traction on the stripper and the skin graft is sutured in place. Thorough hemostasis of the tract in the subcutaneous tissue and of the bed of excision of the stasis area is required to prevent a hematoma from forming under the newly implanted graft.

A continuous suture is used to complete the implantation of the graft after it has been trimmed to occupy the defect with proper tension and held in the desired position with a few interrupted sutures placed around its edge.

[Stasis ulcer excision and skin graft *continued on page 206.*]

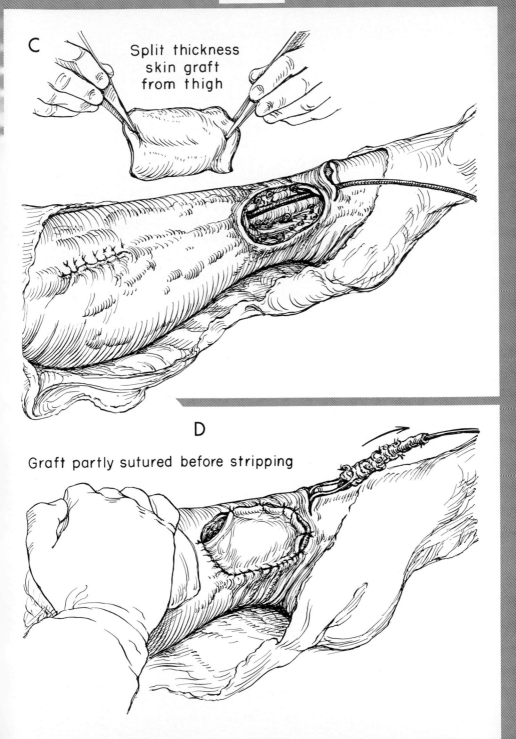

PLATE 67

C

Split thickness
skin graft
from thigh

D

Graft partly sutured before stripping

One area of the graft is left unsutured for careful irrigation, and in many instances the procedure is completed as the circumferential suturing of graft to bed is finished. This is probably desirable only when there is little or no opportunity for any degree of infection, as in those cases in which the ulcer had been healed completely before surgery.

An alternative method is illustrated which may offer significant advantage when the resection is done in the presence of an open ulcer. The graft is perforated in multiple areas (*E*) and is sutured to the bed with interrupted fine sutures (*E* and *F*) to prevent motion and elevation by blood or serum. Further, very small catheters are incorporated in the gauze wadding over the ulcer and under the compression dressing (*G*) in order that an antibiotic solution may be applied topically during the postoperative period.

PLATE 67

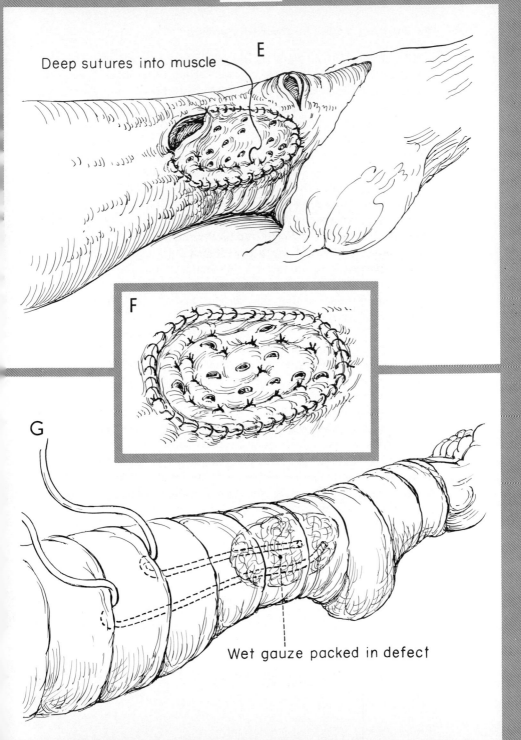

Deep sutures into muscle

E

F

G

Wet gauze packed in defect

Dissection and division of the incompetent perforator channels can be accomplished by one of two techniques. These are (1) the suprafascial identification and division of the offending channels at the points of their perforation of the fascia, or (2) the subfascial approach to the same vessels and their interruption on the underside of the deep fascia of the leg. The suprafascial dissection is performed only in those patients with minimally altered subcutaneous tissue. The subfascial technique is employed in the more common situation in which, as a result of the venous pathology, a considerable amount of subcutaneous fibrosis has already occurred. If the subcutaneous tissues are scarred, it is inappropriate to damage them further by dissection above the fascia, as this will compromise the ability of these tissues to heal during the postoperative period.

The extremity is prepared in its entirety and the foot covered with stockinet or a sterile rubber glove. The incision is placed posterior and parallel to the tibia on the medial calf, extending from the area posterior to the upper margin of the medial malleolus upward to the midcalf level above the stasis change (*A*). Often an area of more advanced stasis change will have to be incised as the surgeon divides the skin, and meticulous technique in handling the cutaneous margins must be employed if healing is to be expected. In the event that the subcutaneous tissues are normal, the perforating veins are identified in this layer, as shown in *B*, and the connecting varicosities excised. Each perforator is ligated at its point of emergence through the deep fascia (*C*).

If the subcutaneous tissues are at all fibrous and abnormal, it is advisable to incise the fascia longitudinally and locate the perforating veins beneath it, as shown in *D*. The fascia is approximated with interrupted catgut sutures and the skin closed with fine Nylon suture material (*E*). The choice of the latter material for the skin closure is based upon its tendency to produce minimal tissue reaction so that it is well tolerated during the period of primary healing, which may be prolonged.

PLATE 68

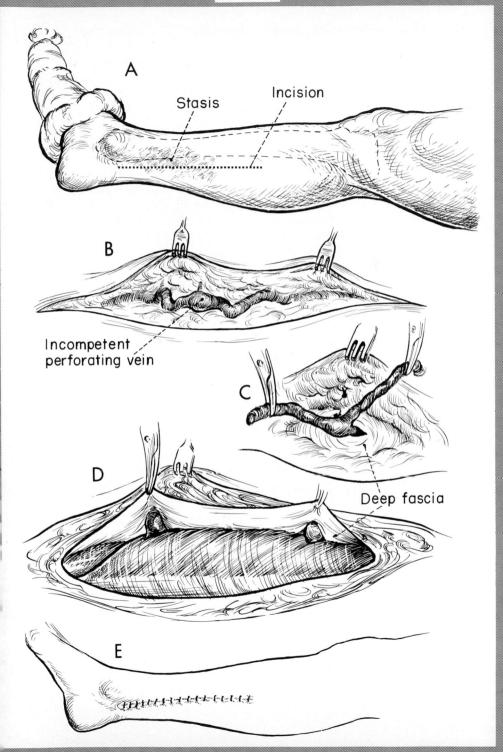

A

Stasis   Incision

B

Incompetent
perforating vein

C

Deep fascia

D

E

Inferior Vena Cava Ligation – Plication

Surgical fenestration or ligation of the inferior vena cava most often is indicated because of the failure of anticoagulant therapy to prevent embolic phenomena or in the presence of a contraindication to anticoagulant therapy in a patient with deep thrombophlebitis. Plate 69, *A* and *B*, depicts the technique.

The right flank incision shown in *A* is used. The layers of the abdominal wall are separated in the direction of their fibers and the retroperitoneal space entered. The inferior vena cava is then encircled, with the ligature placed just distal to the largest available lumbar branch (*B*). The selection of such a point is important because inflow from the branch prevents stasis and thrombosis above the ligature. Fenestration by suture or by clip device may be used as alternative techniques.

Femoral Vein Thrombectomy

Femoral thrombectomy continues to be the subject of reviews and evaluation. The purpose is the immediate reduction of venous insufficiency and the minimizing of postphlebitic disability. Only patients with iliofemoral involvement (nonrecurrent) and/or recent onset of thrombosis should be selected.

A groin incision is made as shown in *A*, using local anesthesia. The femoral vein and its tributaries are exposed, and thrombi are then removed locally from the femoral vein (*C*). Thrombi proximal and distal to the venotomy are removed by balloon catheters (*D*), with the patient performing the Valsalva maneuver during proximal clot extraction. As a prophylaxis against surgically induced embolism, one may elect either to obstruct the inferior vena cava temporarily with a separately inserted balloon catheter or to use direct exposure and control of the inferior vena cava.

Primary repair of the incision in the vein is shown in *E*.

PLATE 69

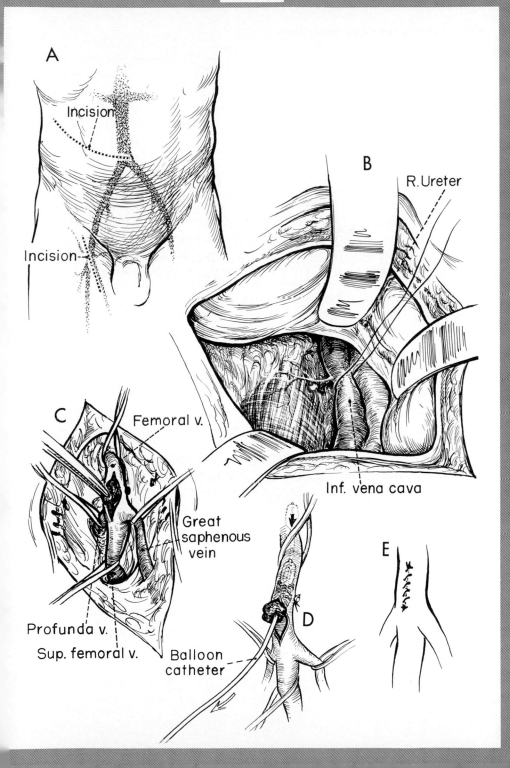

The diagnosis of pulmonary embolism is made on clinical grounds with the assistance of the chest x-ray and electrocardiogram. Usually the diagnosis is confirmed by obtaining a lung scan or pulmonary arteriogram. The majority of patients diagnosed as having such an embolus are best treated by supportive measures plus anticoagulation and in some instances by inferior vena caval interruption. At present, patients selected for pulmonary embolectomy are those who are not likely to survive other therapy and who usually manifest some degree of shock.

The precarious condition of the patient usually requires that cannulation for the heart-lung machine be done before general anesthesia is given and the median sternotomy incision made (*A*). The femoral artery and vein can usually be used, with the jugular vein an alternate if the femoral veins are thrombosed. Anesthesia is then induced with the patient on partial cardiopulmonary by-pass. Administration of anesthesia without such provision may result in total cardiovascular-pulmonary collapse. After the sternum has been split and the pericardium opened, the superior vena cava is cannulated and the pulmonary artery is isolated for incision (*B*). With the superior and inferior vena cava occluded and total cardiopulmonary by-pass established, the pulmonary artery is incised (*C*) and forceps used to withdraw the larger emboli. It may be helpful to compress and milk the lung to express smaller ones. The pulmonary artery is then repaired and the by-pass discontinued.

Prior to the conclusion of the procedure, an extraperitoneal right flank ligation incision is made for plication of the inferior vena cava.

PLATE 70

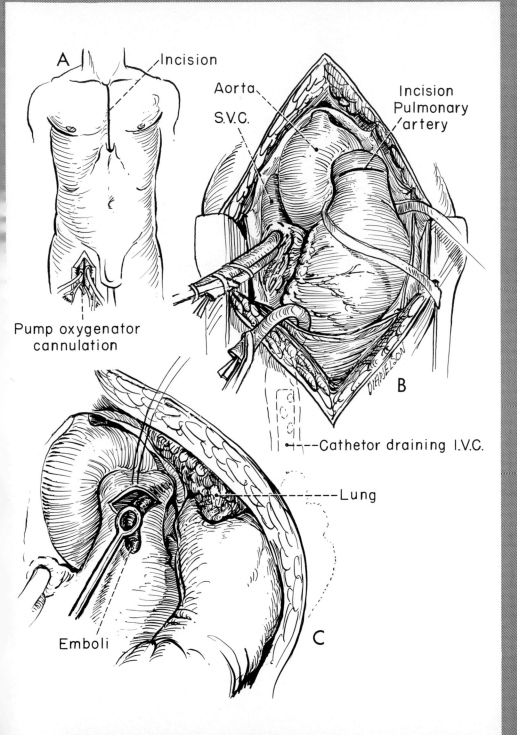

A

Incision

Aorta

S.V.C.

Incision
Pulmonary
artery

Pump oxygenator
cannulation

B

Cathetor draining I.V.C.

Lung

Emboli

C

CHAPTER 13

Portal Hypertension

THE CURRENT CONCEPT of portal hypertension and the adaptation of the Eck fistula to clinical use were first introduced by Whipple in 1945. Portal hypertension is said to exist when the pressure in the portal system exceeds 150–200 mm. of water. There is no question that portal pressure varies from day to day, even in patients with pathologic elevations of such pressure. It is also true that the exact mechanism of production of portal hypertension is not entirely clear. Portal hypertension may exist for many years without the patient's being aware of it. Patients seek treatment because of bleeding from esophageal gastric varices, the presence of hypersplenism, ascites or hepatic failure. The physiologic factors in the development of portal hypertension exist either in obstruction to portal flow in the liver (so-called intrahepatic obstruction) or in obstruction in the portal vein (so-called sub· or prehepatic obstruction). Additional obstruction sites may be at the outlet of the liver in the hepatic veins or venules (Budd-Chiari syndrome). Portal hypertension may be a reflection of chronic heart failure.

In general, most of the patients who are seen with portal hypertension have intrahepatic obstruction or cirrhosis of the liver. One associates extrahepatic obstruction with the younger age group and with portal thrombosis secondary to omphalitis or other cause. The number of children seen with extrahepatic obstruction is limited, whereas the number of adults with cirrhosis is much greater. Patients with cirrhosis vary greatly in clinical appearance — from the wasted, chronically ill alcoholic to the successful executive.

The diagnosis of portal hypertension is usually stimulated by the appearance of the patient with bleeding varices. Varices may be confirmed by barium swallow in about 70 per cent of patients. Esophagoscopy provides the most accurate estimate of the size and extent of esophageal varices, and in competent hands it is a safe method of examination. The differentiation between intra- and extrahepatic obstruction on the basis of laboratory examinations is sometimes difficult, particularly in the cirrhotic with relatively normal liver functions. Given an obvious case of cirrhosis, however, the most reasonable cause of portal hypertension is intrahepatic obstruction due to the cirrhosis. It is true, however, that 5–8 per cent of these patients also have thrombosis of the portal vein.

The appearance of hypersplenism in a child with a large spleen but with normal liver functions draws attention immediately to extrahepatic obstruction. Hypersplenism secondary to long-standing intrahepatic obstruction in the adult is a rather frequent occurrence. More sophisticated methods such as splenoportography will pinpoint the exact site of the obstruction. Splenoportography, in which a long needle or a catheter threaded over a needle is introduced into the spleen and contrast material injected, will visualize the splenic vein and the portal vein and give much information about the status of the portal venous system. In addition, the pressure can be measured. The splenic pulp pressure approximates the true portal pressure. More recently the introduction of catheters through the umbilical vein has provided a method for measuring pressure as well as a site for introduction of contrast material for radiographic visualization. In addition, the cannulation of the umbilical vein has been used as the portal connection for a temporary portal-systemic shunt.

The mechanism for the initiation of the variceal hemorrhage is not clear. Although formerly it was thought to be most often due to peptic acid effect with erosion of the varices, as well as to the effect of rough foods, the lack of findings of peptic esophagitis at the time of surgery of the esophagus has minimized this as a possible cause. Although the changes in the portal pressure may precipitate bleeding, in general the exact cause of the hemorrhage is unknown.

PORTAL HYPERTENSION IN CHILDREN

Portal system obstruction occurs in children predominantly at the portal vein level. It is probably more often due to portal vein thrombosis secondary either to dehydration or to inflammation entering through the venous channels from an omphalitis, usually during the first few days of life. This obstruction produces congestive enlargement of the spleen and secondary hypersplenism with characteristic bone marrow changes and pancytopenia. Ascites occurs less frequently than it does in portal obstruction on the basis of liver disease. The submucous veins of the esophagus enlarge as a part of the collateral system which develops to provide splanchnic venous drainage around the obstruction.

The esophageal collaterals are subject to mechanical tearing and, it is supposed, to occasional erosion in connection with esophagitis. The episodes of bleeding that plague and threaten the affected youngster and the anemia of hypersplenism are indications for surgical therapy. Splenectomy will relieve the hypersplenism but does nothing for the portal hypertension or the esophageal varices except in rare instances in which only the splenic vein was originally involved.

A variety of procedures on the esophagus have been used to remove the source of bleeding. Among these are esophagectomy with jejunal or colonic interposition and direct suture of the varices through the surgically exposed esophagus.

The portacaval anastomosis is often impossible in the child with portal hypertension because the portal vein is virtually absent, being replaced by small collateral veins—the so-called "cavernomatous transformation." Splenorenal anastomosis is most useful if the patient reaches age 8–10 years, at which time the vessels are large enough for a dependable anastomosis.

The more recently developed mesenteric-caval shunt diagramed in Plate 74, C provides a reliable portal-systemic drainage procedure for children whose portal veins are not available.

Ascites

Ascites, rather than bleeding, is the primary problem in some patients with portal hypertension. Etiologic factors in ascites have been subject to much discussion. The effects of osmotic pressure and the redistribution of the albumin in the ascitic fluid have been incriminated. The effects of sodium retention with increased body water secondary to this sodium retention may result in hypoalbuminemia due to dilution as well as in hyponatremia. The marked retention of water also suggests an excess of antidiuretic hormone. Increased aldosterone activity also leads to increased retention of sodium.

The exact mechanism of ascitic fluid formation is not entirely clear. The most important factor, according to many, is the obstruction to the hepatic outflow, namely, the postsinusoidal area in the liver. Fibrosis and regenerating hepatic liver nodules result in obstruction and increasing sinusoidal pressure. The hormonal factors are considered as secondary. Portal hypertension alone does not result in ascites.

The role of the lymphatics is an important one, and the seepage of lymph fluid from the lymphatics to the liver contributes markedly to the production of ascites. The more recent application of decompression of the thoracic duct and alleviation of ascitic fluid formation would tend to support this factor. A portal-systemic shunt, such as side-to-side shunt, for ascites alone is indicated occasionally.

APPROACH TO PORTAL VEIN

Techniques for end-to-side, the most common, and side-to-side portacaval shunts are shown in Plates 72 and 73. Although formerly a thoracoabdominal approach was used to this problem, in recent years all such shunts have been done through a subcostal incision, such as that shown in *A*. The liver is retracted cephalad (*B*) and the duodenum may be dissected in a typical Kocher maneuver. Here the bleeding may be far more extensive than one usually sees in this avascular maneuver and may require multiple ligations of tiny collaterals.

The common duct is identified and dissected free, and the dissection is directed posterior to the common duct toward the portal vein. The sheath of peritoneal reflection about the portal vein, the anterior boundary of the foramen of Winslow, may be grasped and used as a holder while the portal vein is dissected by sharp dissection with scissors as well as by finger dissection in order to encircle the portal vein. A small coronary vein branch on the left side of the portal vein may be encountered, and this may need ligating. In addition, a small branch is often encountered superiorly near the division of the portal vein. The large node present at the junction of the common duct of the duodenum may or may not be dissected free, but in most cases removing it facilitates the proper turning of the vein downward when an end-to-side shunt is done. It is dissected free and multiple ligatures taken because of the collateral present here, as shown in *C*. In *D*, the portal vein has been completely dissected free, and in this particular instance a portion of the caudate lobe has been dissected. This is necessary in a certain number of cases.

[End-to-side portacaval shunt *on page 222.*]

PLATE 71

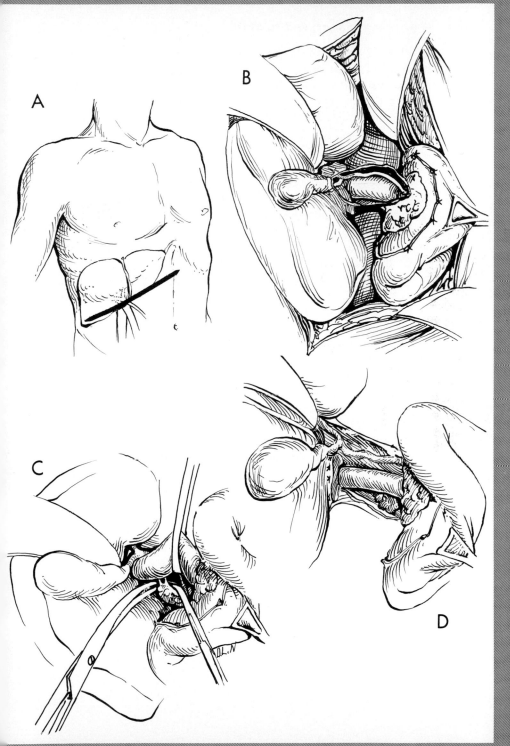

Plate 72 shows the technical details of the end-to-side portacaval shunt. Following dissection of the portal vein (Plate 71), the vein is ligated as high as possible with a heavy silk suture (*A*), and a vascular clamp is placed across it proximally. The inferior vena cava has been dissected free and is shown posteriorly. It is important to dissect the vena cava extensively to permit easy application of the partially occluding clamp. This is particularly true on the medial and left sides of the vena cava. In *B*, the portal vein is transected. This is done in more or less of an oblique way, because when the vein is turned down to join the vena cava, the angle is such that obliquity of the portal vein makes for a more satisfactory anastomosis. The clamp on the portal vein is released temporarily to flush out blood and to be sure that there are no clots present. In *C*, a partially occluding clamp has been placed on the vena cava, and the dotted line shows the line of excision of a portion of the anterior wall. The clamp is placed more or less on the medial or left anterior aspect of the vena cava so that the portal vein will lie in such a fashion that it will not kink. The somewhat rectangular excision results in a more circular hole for the anastomosis.

D illustrates the end-to-side shunt. This is done with two 5–0 continuous silk or Teflon-Dacron sutures, the back wall being done first from above downward and then the anterior row being completed. An alternate method is to use everting continuous horizontal mattress sutures; this is somewhat more difficult technically on the back wall, but does eliminate suture material in the lumen of the shunt. In *E*, the completed end-to-side shunt is shown.

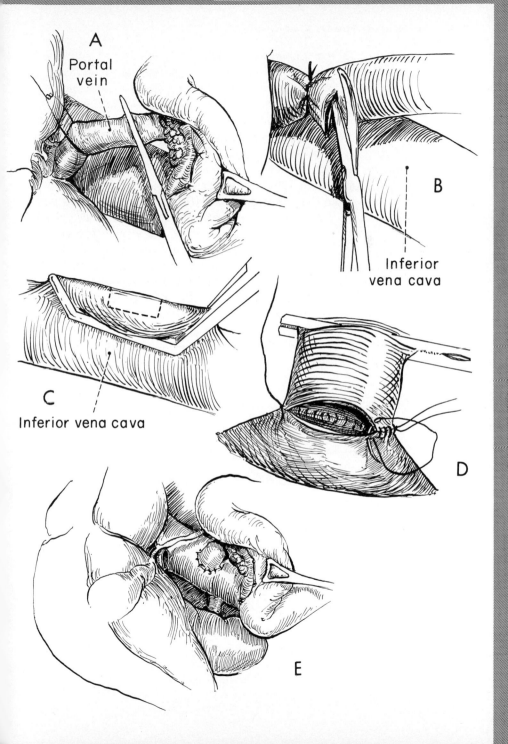

PLATE 72

A

Portal vein

B

Inferior vena cava

C

Inferior vena cava

D

E

In Plate 73 the technical details of a side-to-side shunt are shown. The preliminary dissection of the portal vein is done as in Plate 71. The ideal anatomic situation for side-to-side shunt is that in which the distance between the portal vein and the anterior aspect of the vena cava is not too great. On rare occasions a graft has been used to bridge this distance, end-to-side to the side of the portal vein on its posterior aspect and end-to-side to the anterior wall of the vena cava. If a graft is used, it must be a large-lumen synthetic graft (in the neighborhood of 14 mm.) to avoid closure.

In *A* are shown the dissected portal vein and the vena cava posteriorly. The duodenum and pancreas are retracted on the right. Nontraumatic clamps are placed across the portal vein proximally and distally (*B*). An elliptic excision of a portion of the posterior wall of the portal vein is shown in *C*, and a similar excision is made of the anterior wall of the vena cava after application of the partially occluding clamp (*D*). The portal vein has been rotated to the left and anastomosis is started in the usual manner with two 5–0 sutures (*D*). An over-and-over running suture is used posteriorly and then anteriorly, as shown in *E*. The completed side-to-side shunt is shown in *F*.

PLATE 73

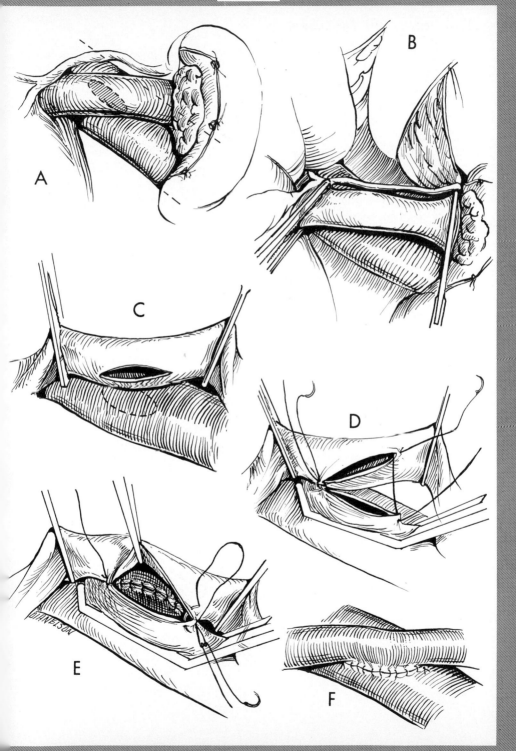

Other types of shunts less frequently used are shown in this plate. In *A*, the classical splenorenal anastomosis is shown completed. The spleen is removed, the splenic artery is ligated and the splenic vein is preserved with as much length as possible. Meticulous dissection of the splenic vein is accomplished as it passes medially along the upper border of the pancreas; many of the tiny branches need to be ligated. A partially occluding clamp is applied to the renal vein and a standard end-to-side shunt done with continuous 5 – 0 suture.

B shows a more recent application of a so-called selective portal decompression, as advocated by Warren. Here the spleen is left in and the distal splenic vein is turned down to the renal vein. This type of shunt diverts the portal blood flow from the left upper quadrant of the abdomen and the critical esophageal-gastric area, producing decompression of that area. It supposedly is accompanied by a lower incidence of ammonia intoxication than more complete diversion of portal venous flow.

In *C* is shown the mesenteric vein-inferior vena caval shunt advocated by Marion and Clatworthy. The distal vena cava is ligated and the end of the inferior vena cava turned and anastomosed to the side of the superior mesenteric vein. This shunt is particularly valuable, as mentioned before, in very young children in whom there is extrahepatic obstruction of the portal vein and the splenic vein is entirely too small for a splenorenal shunt. This shunt may also be used in adults when extrahepatic obstruction is present, particularly when a splenorenal shunt has failed.

PLATE 74

A

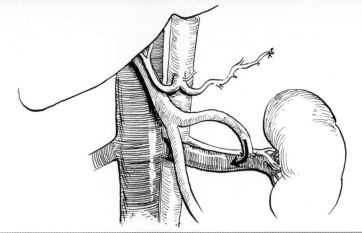

B

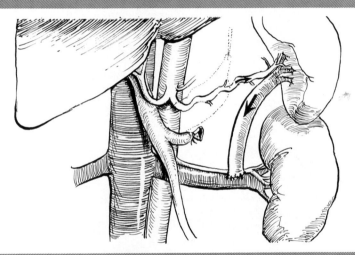

C

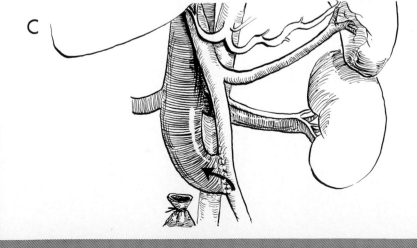

The Heart and Great Vessels

CHAPTER 14

Introduction

FEW EXAMPLES of the application of physiologic principles to a broad clinical problem parallel the development of corrective surgery on the heart and great vessels. The clarification of the hemodynamics involved in the pathologic conditions and the progressive availability of corrective surgical techniques have been mutually stimulating to groups of surgeons and physiologists working in the field. Concurrently, and as a result, there has been a remarkable refinement of understanding of the clinical features and diagnosis of cardiac lesions. In this atmosphere, corrective surgery has progressed rapidly through successive phases. The earliest of these is represented by the correction of patent ductus arteriosus and coarctation of the aorta, examples of extracardiac anomalies. Procedures then became available for intracardiac surgery in which the corrective manipulations were carried out without direct visualization and without interruption of cardiac function. This phase was represented by mitral commissurotomy, pulmonary valvulotomy for congenital stenosis, transventricular aortic valvulotomy and a variety of procedures used in repair of interatrial septal defects. Direct exposure of structures within the heart for their repair was first afforded by the use of general body hypothermia, which permits interruption of the circulation for limited periods. The longer time required for the repair of more complicated defects was obtained by the clinical application of extracorporeal gas exchange in the form of the heart-lung machine, permitting cardiac by-pass.

Improvements directed toward obtaining a more quiet and dry field then emerged. Cardiac arrest induced by the administration of potassium or acetylcholine or simply by interruption of coronary circulation provided a quiet heart but was found to be damaging to the heart muscle. To a limited degree, reduction of the temperature of the myocardium during periods of interruption of coronary circulation is considered an optimum technique in many centers.

As the confinements of exposure, time and a quiet field have been overcome, the limitations to the success of repair imposed by the severity of the pathologic processes present the increasingly important challenge. This is particularly true for the surgical repair of acquired valvular disease, in which the damage is often so extensive that reconstruction using the patient's own tissues becomes impossible. Whereas the development of prosthetic replacements for use in a nonfunctioning situation, such as large defects in the septa, was relatively simple, prostheses which must function, as is the case with valve structures, were more difficult to provide. The prosthetics currently available for replacement of the aortic, mitral and tricuspid valves are the result of close cooperation in development between technologists in several fields and surgeons. The results of their use indicate that confidence in them is not misplaced. Valves incorporating new features appear at frequent intervals, indicating that we are still in a phase of problem solving, even though our present prostheses are very advanced. Their design resists the formation of thrombi which could detach and cause peripheral artery emboli. The ability of the tissues to attach by scar infiltration to the artificial valve ring has been well demonstrated and is only rarely inadequate. Nevertheless, the aggressive use of prostheses and of homologous valves, which offer another approach to the problem, continues to be tempered by critical comparison of the prognosis of the patient if he is not offered surgical treatment with that obtained if a replacement is done.

This section on the heart and great vessels will deal primarily with procedures that are well established. A few which are no longer much used will be included, either because they represent important steps in development of cardiac surgery or because their use has been reported in the surgical literature and the results are still being observed. Finally, some operations are included because they represent the expanding horizon of the field.

Indications and contraindications for the various procedures are not within the scope of this volume. The selection for surgery of patients in all categories, however, is subject to generalization which proves to be accurate whenever it is specifically applied. Surgical decision depends on evaluation of these several factors:

1. The course which may be anticipated if surgery is withheld.

2. The degree to which this course will be favorably influenced if surgery is accomplished successfully.

3. The present risk.

4. The likelihood that a better procedure will be evolved in a period of time not too long for the patient to wait.

Evaluation of these factors will result in a strong indication for surgery when normal function can be restored at little risk even though the lesion is one unlikely soon to have serious consequences. This opinion applies most strongly in conditions such as patent ductus, coarctation and interatrial septal defect. There is uncertainty about the course of patients with mild forms of interventricular septal defect which centers about the question of development of pulmonary vascular changes. Differences in interpretation of the first factor, therefore, result in different approaches to the treatment of this lesion in various clinics.

The second factor, which reflects the restoration which will result from successful surgery, includes the possibility of recurrence. This factor applies particularly to stenotic changes in the mitral valve secondary to rheumatic fever. The demonstrated hazard of recurrence after mitral commissurotomy requires that the patient with mitral stenosis have significant and real cardiac limitations before surgery is done. Risk, the third factor, diminishes with experience. It is often found to be profoundly affected by the severity of the heart disease which quantifies the need for surgery. The policy of any cardiac surgical center in the matter of balancing need with risk in applying surgical therapy largely determines its statistics in terms of morbidity, mortality and the quality of results.

CHAPTER 15

General Techniques in Surgery

A HIGH DEGREE of accuracy of preoperative diagnosis is required for the efficient repair of a cardiac defect. Fortunately, this is provided in the majority of cases by physiologic and x-ray studies. However, the first stage of each surgical procedure is one of examination to evaluate the preoperative diagnosis. As in the preliminary exploration of the abdomen before carrying out the planned procedure, this is most efficient if a routine of observation and measurement is followed. The major points in the exploration include the following:

1. Relationship in position and in size of the major vessels at the cardiac base.

2. Size of the atria and their color as it reflects the content of arterial or venous blood.

3. Distribution, size and consistency of the coronary arteries.

4. Ventricular size and muscular consistency and the composition of the apex by left or right ventricle or both.

5. Search for a persistent left superior vena cava and palpation for an unsuspected patent ductus.

6. Palpation and localization of thrills over the heart and great vessels.

7. Intracardiac palpation through either atrium to determine anatomic details of septal defects or the severity of damage of atrioventricular valves.

8. Pressure measurements in appropriate locations.

Bilateral anterior thoracotomy involving transection of the sternum, the incision most used in the earliest work in open heart surgery, provides the broadest exposure of the heart and basal vessels. This incision, however, provided exposure at great expense in postoperative pain, immobility of the chest and consequent postoperative pulmonary complications. Unilateral thoracotomy and anterior mediastinotomy involving longitudinal splitting of the sternum have largely replaced it.

The relationship of the circulatory viscera to various levels and positions of incisions in the right chest is suggested in *A*. A right thoracotomy provides exposure for isolation of the venae cavae and for operations on the tricuspid and mitral valves through the right and left atria, respectively, and on the interatrial septum. Cardiac operations through the right chest offer the best exposure when done through the fourth interspace or through the bed of the resected fourth rib. The incision is usually made anterior and lateral, there being no need for a high posterior extension.

Incisions in the left chest are used for operations on the aorta and the ductus and for blind manipulations of the mitral, aortic and sometimes the pulmonary valves. Cardiopulmonary by-pass can be established through the left chest by cannulation of the pulmonary artery or right ventricle, plus obstruction of the pulmonary artery. This method of pump connection is useful in operations on the mitral valve and left ventricular chamber or wall. An anterior fourth interspace incision on the left exposes the left atrium for digital manipulation of the mitral valve. It will be noted from the relationship shown in *B* that an anterolateral incision in the fifth interspace provides essentially the same exposure of the atrium, while at the same time permitting introduction of a dilator through the apex of the left ventricle for the addition of mechanical force in opening the mitral valve. An incision in the fourth interspace or through the bed of the resected fourth rib exposes the body of the ventricles for such an operation as pericardiectomy. If a fourth interspace incision on the left side is extended across the sternum into the anterior right thorax for a short distance, the pericardiectomy is more easily completed around the base of the heart and in the atrioventricular grooves.

[Thoracotomy incisions *continued on page 236.*]

PLATE 75

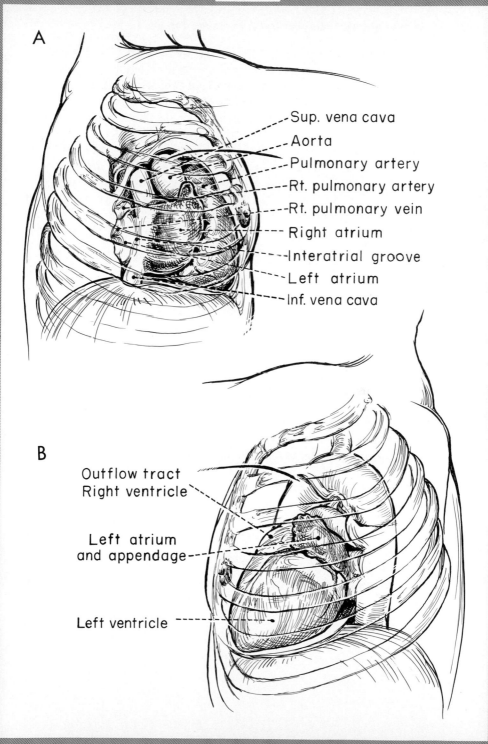

A

Sup. vena cava
Aorta
Pulmonary artery
Rt. pulmonary artery
Rt. pulmonary vein
Right atrium
Interatrial groove
Left atrium
Inf. vena cava

B

Outflow tract
Right ventricle

Left atrium
and appendage

Left ventricle

The anterior exposure of the mediastinal structures afforded by an anterior sternum-splitting incision approximates that of a bilateral anterior thoracotomy and avoids the pulmonary complications that occur following the latter. One of the principal disadvantages of the sternum-splitting incision is the great frequency with which keloids form in the skin over the sternum. Also, if a patent ductus is incidentally encountered, control is much more difficult through the sternal incision than through a bilateral thoracotomy.

The incision for midline sternotomy is usually made vertically in the midline of the chest. To avoid extending the skin incision up to the sternal notch, another incision is made transversely at the upper end at the level of the second rib (C). The lower end of the midline skin incision is extended for a distance into the epigastrium below the xiphoid process to avoid any restrictions in this region in lateral retraction of the two halves of the sternum.

The skin and subcutaneous tissue are elevated from the sternum only at the upper extremity where this is necessary to expose the sternal notch. The periosteum of the sternum (D) is incised in the midline of the sternum and elevated for a short distance on each side. The sternum is then cut longitudinally, using a vibrating saw (E). During longitudinal section of the sternum it is important to cool the blade of the rapidly vibrating instrument to prevent damage to bone by heat. Saline irrigation is effective in this regard.

After the bone has been incised, the soft tissues of the mediastinum are dissected bluntly from its undersurface on each side (F). A strong fibrous band will be palpable traversing the retrosternal tissues at the sternal notch. This condensation is the interclavicular ligament and it must be cut with scissors to allow the upper ends of the divided sternum to separate.

A self-retaining rib spreader is then placed transversely in the sternotomy wound (G), and the pericardium is incised anteriorly in the area free from pleura. Superiorly the thymus gland is elevated from the pericardium and the latter structure is incised behind it. An attempt is made to avoid opening either pleural cavity at this point in the operation, although at the time of closure it may be judged desirable to provide drainage of the pericardium into either pleural cavity.

PLATE 75

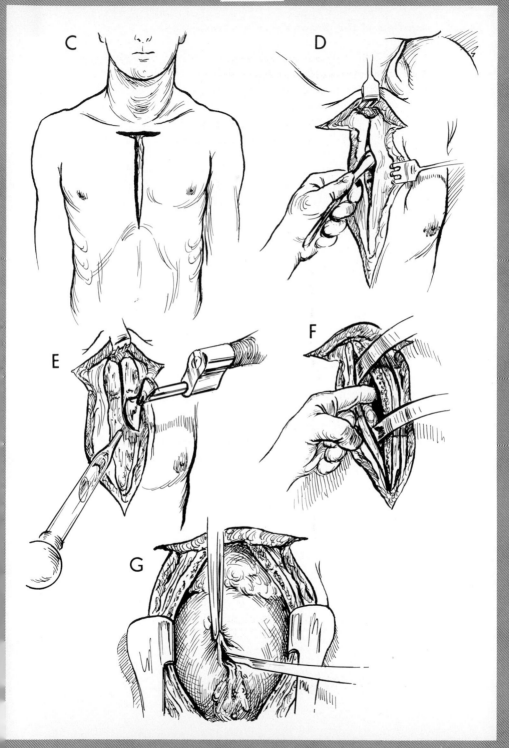

The isolation and encirclement with control tapes of the superior and inferior venae cavae, pulmonary artery and aorta are steps in preparation for operations utilizing either hypothermia and temporary inflow occlusion or cardiopulmonary by-pass with a pump-oxygenator. Many of these operations are done through a median sternotomy, illustrated in this plate.

Encirclement of the superior vena cava is most easily accomplished and is done first because the tape can then be used to retract the vessel during isolation of the aorta. The dissection starts from within the pericardium. With the superior vena cava retracted laterally, a very small incision is made in the visceral pericardium at its reflection on the medial aspect of the cava at the superior border of the right pulmonary artery. A curved hemostat introduced through this point and directed laterally behind the cava is then easily pushed through the pericardial reflection on the lateral side of the vessel. A tape placed in its grasp (*A*) is drawn through to encircle the vessel.

Separation of the pulmonary. artery and aorta is begun in the visceral pericardium covering their adjacent anterior surfaces. After the pericardium is incised the dissection down between the vessels (*B*) is carried out under good visualization to avoid damaging the left coronary artery if it should have an abnormally high origin from the aorta. This line of dissection is directed as much as possible downward toward the cardiac base as it progresses toward the posterior aspect of the vessels in order that the transverse pericardial sinus is entered at a point below the origin of the right pulmonary artery. When the transverse sinus has been entered, tapes may be passed individually around aorta and pulmonary artery using the same tract.

Only the beginning of the dissection behind the inferior vena cava can be done under direct vision. The actual passage of the instrument behind the vena cava (*C*) is guided by the thumb and finger of the left hand placed around the vessel. The posterior wall of the vein is palpated by compressing it between the fingers.

Encirclement of all the vessels is shown in *D* at a stage in which preparation for operations of either classification is completed.

[Isolation of great vessels *continued on page 240.*]

PLATE 76

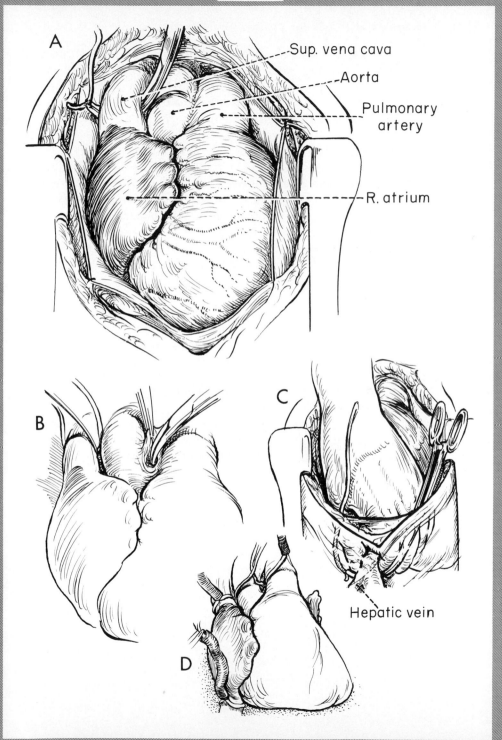

A

Sup. vena cava

Aorta

Pulmonary artery

R. atrium

B

C

D

Hepatic vein

Encirclement of the pulmonary artery for its temporary occlusion during repair of right-sided defects may present some problem in instances of left-to-right shunt in which the pulmonary artery is extremely large. In such cases, if it is not anticipated that there will be need for individual obstruction of the aorta, the pulmonary artery obstruction can be accomplished by the method illustrated in *E* and *F*, which does not require a dissection between the aorta and pulmonary artery. In *E*, the position of the tapes previously placed around the superior vena cava and inferior vena cava is shown. A tape has been passed through the transverse pericardial sinus behind the great vessels. During cardiopulmonary by-pass, with the aorta under pressure from the heart-lung machine and the right heart decompressed through an atriotomy or ventriculotomy, a proper amount of tension placed on this tape will compress the pulmonary artery against the aorta without embarrassing the circulation through the latter vessel.

Another use of the transverse pericardial sinus is illustrated in *G* and *H*. The purpose of this maneuver is to encircle the enlarged pulmonary artery without danger of damage to the right pulmonary artery in the process. In *G* a tape is passed around the aorta, taking advantage of a dissection between the pulmonary artery and aorta which enters the transverse pericardial sinus posteriorly in relation to the aorta. If the free end of the tape is then passed in reverse through the pericardial sinus, the pulmonary artery will be effectively encircled without a dissection having to be made along its medial surface in relation to the origin of the right branch.

PLATE 76

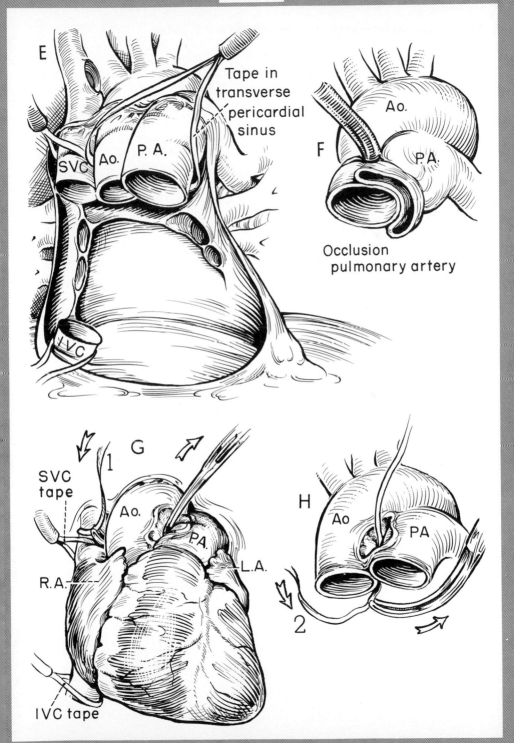

E

Tape in transverse pericardial sinus

SVC Ao. P. A.

IVC

F

Ao.

P.A.

Occlusion pulmonary artery

SVC tape

1 G

Ao.

P. A.

R.A.

L.A.

IVC tape

H

Ao

PA

2

During cardiopulmonary by-pass using a heart-lung machine, blood is collected through two catheters, one placed in each vena cava. Tapes placed about each vein at its junction with the right atrium, as already described, can then be drawn up to direct all blood to the equipment. There are several methods of introducing the flexible plastic catheters. The superior vena cava is cannulated through the right atrial appendage or some other site in the wall of the atrium. The inferior vena cava can be cannulated through the appendage, through an opening made in the atrium or from below by way of the common femoral or iliac vein. The last method is of particular use when it is necessary to start a partial perfusion to support a failing circulation before the chest is opened. In such cases early femoral artery cannulation is also done.

In *A*, the right atrial appendage has been incised after a heavy silk pursestring suture was placed around its base. The catheter tip slips through this opening and is easily directed into the inferior vena cava. The locations of two pursestringed openings with the catheters in place are shown in *B*.

It is sometimes convenient to introduce both catheters through the same right atrial opening, usually in the appendage. This single opening is partitioned for double cannulation (*C*) by a suture passed through the two sides at about the center of the atriotomy. This suture is later tied (*D*) to prevent leaks between the catheters which have been placed in the appropriate venae cavae.

Cannulation of the inferior vena cava through the femoral vein is diagrammed in *E*. The catheter is passed well into the inferior vena cava, where the size of the lumen of the vessel will facilitate drainage. The vein is easily repaired later.

Arterial cannulation for return of oxygenated blood from the heart-lung machine utilizes either the femoral or the iliac artery and, infrequently, the left subclavian artery. It is convenient to expose both the common femoral artery and vein (*F*) for arterial return and inferior vena caval drainage, respectively, through one incision. It is desirable that the artery be cannulated first to avoid a period of venous engorgement in the extremity which would result from occluding the vein before the artery.

PLATE 77

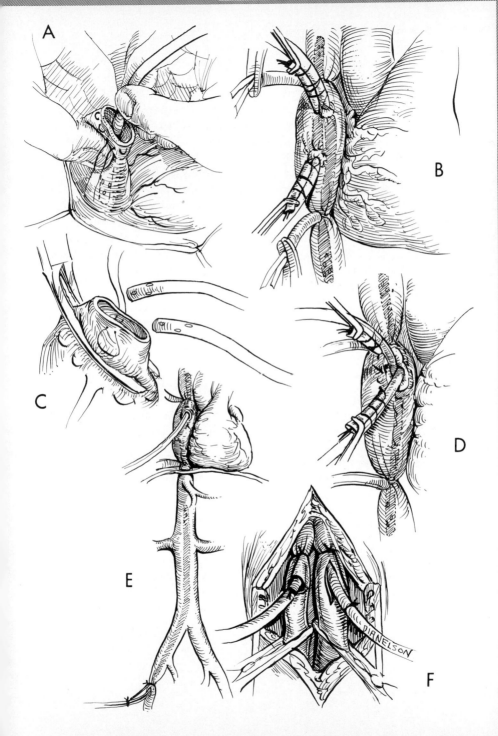

Separate perfusion of the coronary arteries with oxygenated blood from the heart-lung machine makes possible direct operative work on the aortic valve without subjecting the myocardium to anoxia and without necessarily using hypothermia. Undiminished myocardial activity can be maintained during a prolonged period of cardiopulmonary by-pass. If it is desired, local myocardial hypothermia can be induced quickly by cooling the coronary circuit blood, and the coronary perfusion can be discontinued when cold arrest occurs. An immobile heart is obtainable during coronary perfusion at normal temperature also by using a small galvanic current applied to the ventricular wall. This induces ventricular fibrillation and is applied when regular ventricular contractions are considered a disadvantage. Coronary perfusion also is available for reconstructions of the ascending aorta in which transection of the aorta near the aortic valve ring is required.

The method of introducing the cannulas through which the coronary blood supply is maintained is illustrated in this plate in a case of aortic stenosis. Exposure is through a median sternotomy. In *A*, the superior vena cava has been cannulated through the right femoral vein. Each coronary cannula is supplied with oxygenated blood by an individual small roller pump. Each coronary pump circuit is monitored by a pressure meter, and the flow rate is adjusted to keep the pressure at about a normal mean arterial pressure. Rapid increase in the pressure reading usually is a signal that the coronary circuit is occluded. The aorta is cross-clamped and the customary hockey-stick-shaped incision is outlined.

The completed aortic incision is shown in *B* with the diseased aortic valve exposed. The left coronary orifice is located and cannulated with a flexible plastic tube with an expansion near its top (*C*). A suture is passed as a sling through the aortic wall to secure it in the orifice. The suture is threaded through a 2 – 3 in. length of rubber tube which is clamped over the suture after it is drawn tight, as shown in *D*. *E* shows the right coronary artery similarly cannulated.

PLATE 78

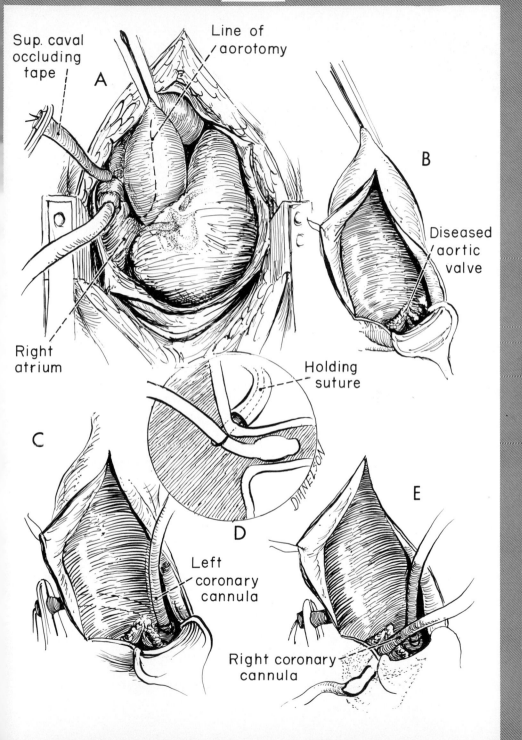

Sup. caval occluding tape

Line of aorotomy

A

B

Diseased aortic valve

Right atrium

Holding suture

C

D

E

Left coronary cannula

Right coronary cannula

DH NELSON

CHAPTER **16**

Surgery
of the Great Vessels

THIS CHAPTER will deal with congenital deformities of
the aorta and only indirectly involves pulmonary artery surgery.
Such lesions of the pulmonary artery which are certainly amenable
to surgery are aneurysm and pulmonary embolism. Pulmonary
aneurysm, a rare lesion, has not been considered to carry nearly
the hazard to life that accompanies systemic aneurysm, and instances of its repair are practically unknown. Pulmonary embolectomy (Plate 70) is more and more frequently done. Its indications
are not yet firmly established except in extreme situations in which
recovery without it is unlikely, and in these a worthwhile salvage
rate is attained. Reconstructive surgery for congenital anomalies of
the aorta, on the other hand, is most satisfactory in that a normal
circulation is almost routinely produced.

The least imposing of these lesions for repair is the common
form of patent ductus treated in childhood. There would seem to
be little probability of error in diagnosis of this lesion. However,
except in experienced hands, a significant percentage of those relatively rare lesions which may be misdiagnosed as patent ductus
may be missed clinically. The surgeon is then in the position of
failing to find the lesions for which his incision was planned, and
judgment will often dictate a second, later procedure. Obviously, a
definitive diagnostic procedure such as retrograde aortography
would prevent this added danger to the patient. It is equally evident that aortography is not routinely necessary as a preliminary to
repair of patent ductus when the diagnostic personnel (surgeon,

cardiologist and pediatrician) are sensitive to the features of an individual case which cast any doubt on the diagnosis. The lesions apt to be misleading are coronary artery malformation, chest wall arteriovenous fistula, pulmonary arteriovenous fistula, aorticopulmonary window, ruptured sinus of valvular aneurysm and ventricular septal defect with prolapse of an aortic cusp. All have some clinical aspects in common with patent ductus but also have characteristics which are adequate for differentiation.

Coarctation similarly requires careful individualization in extension of ordinary clinical evaluation to include angiography. The variations in the anatomy of coarctations are broad, but those which are of disturbing concern to the surgeon are rare. Hypoplasia of the aortic arch and coarctation proximal to the left subclavian artery or even the left carotid are the important examples.

Angiography is an absolute requirement for planning the surgical relief of vascular ring anomalies of the arch and related conditions. The advance information gained leads to economy of dissection and to avoidance of inadvertent interference with essential blood flow by division of the ring at an inappropriate point.

Of the anomalies to be considered, only that of aorticopulmonary window requires the planned use of cardiopulmonary by pass. However, in all such repairs the surgeon must be prepared to interrupt the aortic flow by cross-clamping, either as a planned step or as an emergency measure. The greatest danger arises from the strain placed on the left ventricle. Although the administration of a rapidly acting ganglion-blocking agent diminishes this, most surgeons would agree that partial cardiac by-pass is the optimum protection. The two ways in which this may be done are (1) direct pumping of blood from the left atrium to a femoral artery and (2) collecting of blood from the inferior vena cava and pumping it into a femoral artery after passing it through an oxygenator. Clamping the aorta in the presence of a coarctation produces little or no change in either peripheral resistance or blood supply to tissues. There is, however, major disturbance in both of these when clamping is needed in the course of surgery on an aorta not the site of congenital occlusion.

Exposure of the left thoracic cavity for repair of a patent ductus is provided by an anterolateral third interspace incision in infants and children and by a large fourth interspace incision in adults. With the left lung displaced anteriorly and downward, a general view of the distal aortic arch and the mediastinum is obtained (*A*). The structures lie in their normal positions. A slight dilatation of the aorta just beyond the left subclavian artery may or may not be present. A thrill is palpated in the mediastinal tissues in front of and medial to the aorta in the position of the pulmonary artery. Its point of maximum intensity is indicated by the * on the figure.

A single long incision in the mediastinal pleura extending along the anterior surface of the aorta up onto the proximal subclavian artery exposes the front wall of the aorta. The plane of dissection should be directly on the walls of these vessels to avoid the need of time-consuming redissection in the same area. The dissection is continued, encircling the aorta above and below the level of the patent ductus, which becomes visible early during the exposure (*B*). During this stage, the vagus nerve and its recurrent laryngeal branch are visualized. Ordinarily they are allowed to remain adherent to the undersurface of the anterior portion of the mediastinal pleura, but it may be important on occasion to encircle the vagus nerve with a narrow tape to keep it out of harm's way. During exposure of the medial wall of the aorta distal to the ductus a bronchial artery is often encountered. It should be ligated and cut to avoid its being torn by indirect traction later in the operation. With control of the aorta above and below the origin of the ductus, the dissection along the anterior surface of the ductus is continued, identifying a pocket of pericardium (*C*) which extends down over the pulmonary artery and the ductus in this region. This dissection is best carried out with fine sharp scissors, cutting strands of tissue which come under tension when traction is applied with fine thumb forceps. As the pericardial extension is freed and elevated, the anterior and lateral wall of the pulmonary artery is visualized and cleared.

[Division and suture of patent ductus arteriosus *continued on page 250.*]

PLATE 79

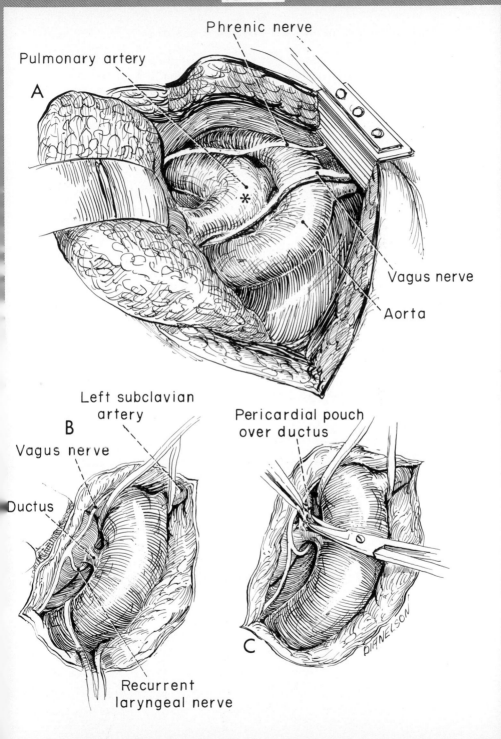

Phrenic nerve

Pulmonary artery

A

*

Vagus nerve

Aorta

Left subclavian
artery

B

Vagus nerve

Ductus

Pericardial pouch
over ductus

C

Recurrent
laryngeal nerve

DIRNELSON

The posterior dissection is carried out until it is possible to palpate a condensation of tissue in the region of the posterior aspect of the pulmonary end of the ductus. This tissue extends from the pulmonary artery to the left main bronchus and limits the mobilization of the pulmonary end of the ductus. This is palpated (*D*) by a finger placed behind the aorta, which is elevated by the two tapes previously placed about it. The tissue must be divided for safe application of the clamp on the pulmonary end of the lesion. This is done, as shown in *E*, as much as possible under direct vision rather than by blunt dissection.

The clamps are applied in such a way as to leave a maximum length of ductus between them (*F*). The aortic clamp is placed near, or even slightly on, the wall of the aorta. If the pulmonary artery pressure is normal, the pulmonary clamp may be placed on the pulmonary artery wall as well. The ductus is then divided all at once if it is of good length. If it is short, it is perhaps better to incise part of the way and to begin each suture line before the rest of the structure is cut. Each suture line is usually placed in two layers (*G* and *H*), the aortic side being repaired first. The first layer is a continuous mattress suture. The second is an over-and-over suture in the cut end of the ductus. The procedure is repeated on the pulmonary side (*I* and *J*). The completed procedure is seen in *K*.

After placement of the sutures it is important on both the aortic and pulmonary sides to remove the ductus clamp in a way such that it does not, in being gradually opened, scrape across the suture line. Rather, as it is released, it is better to push the blades of the clamp against the vessel concerned. The small amount of bleeding that sometimes occurs from suture holes or from the sutured end is controlled by light gauze pressure.

The mediastinal pleura is approximated loosely to diminish adhesions between the lung and the operated surface.

[Division and suture of patent ductus arteriosus *continued on page 252.*]

PLATE 79

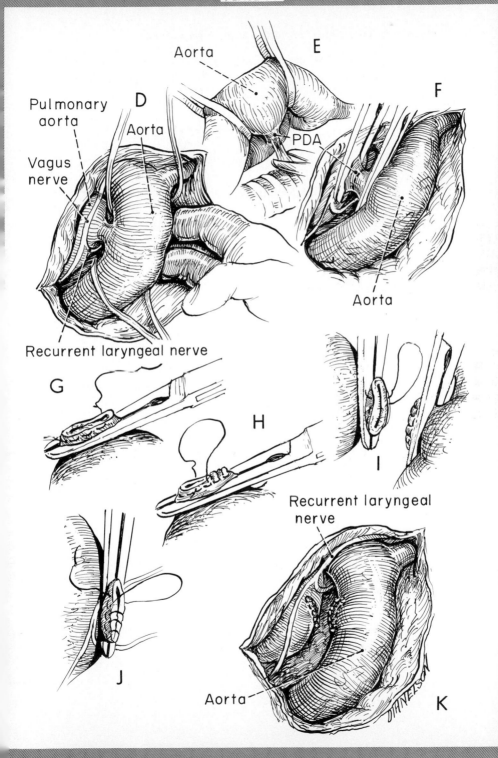

Aorta

E

Pulmonary
aorta

D

Aorta

PDA

F

Vagus
nerve

Aorta

Recurrent laryngeal nerve

G

H

I

Recurrent laryngeal
nerve

J

Aorta

K

DANELSON

Some variation in clamp application may be necessary when a very short, broad ductus is found. One such variation involves the use of a Potts-Smith clamp on the aorta to control the aortic end of the ductus at its base. The aortic wall is used in closure of that end of the ductus, leaving the entire short structure for the pulmonary closure. This technique is particularly desirable when pulmonary hypertension is present and the pulmonary artery is thin walled and fragile.

In addition to complete exposure of the patent ductus arteriosus, the upper one or two pairs of intercostal arteries must be divided (*L*) to give room for application of the Potts-Smith clamp. The clamp is placed around the aorta (*M*) so that its superior and inferior jaws come down on the wall of the aorta adjacent to the ductus. The pulmonary side of the ductus is clamped with a suitable toothed arterial clamp. The Potts clamp, because of its thin construction, has some advantage in this application.

Inasmuch as this method is usually used because of some apprehension as to the strength of the pulmonary artery, the pulmonary artery side of the ductus would ordinarily be repaired first after division (*N*). Thereafter, the aorta is closed (*O*) with, in this instance, a simple over-and-over suture in place of the two-layer closure.

PLATE 79

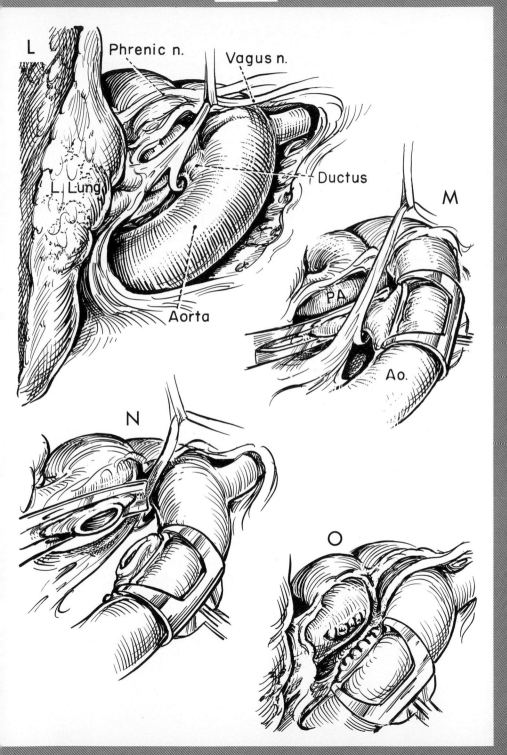

L

Phrenic n.   Vagus n.

L. Lung

Ductus

M

Aorta

PA

Ao.

N

O

Repair of a patent ductus arteriosus in an adult is complicated when enlargement of the adjacent vessels has shortened the lesion and when the ductus and adjacent vessels can be expected to be significantly involved with arteriosclerosis. Preparations for surgery may well include provision for cross-clamping the thoracic aorta to facilitate repair. For a brief period of cross-clamping, reducing the patient's body temperature is adequate. The effects of the increase in peripheral arterial resistance are diminished by using a prompt-acting potent vasodilator.

Another method of compensating for a period of thoracic aortic occlusion is mechanical by-pass of blood from the left atrium to the femoral artery. The left atrium is exposed through a pericardial incision made anterior to the left phrenic nerve with the left lung retracted posteriorly. A pursestring suture is placed around the base of the left auricular appendage (*A* and *B*), and a plastic catheter with adequate perforations near its end is introduced into the atrium (*C*) and brought out through the chest wound. It is passed through a suitable pump of occlusive type and then connected to a cannula which is inserted into the femoral artery. The patient is heparinized.

As the aorta is clamped, blood is pumped from the left atrium to the femoral artery at a rate such that the central aortic root pressure remains constant, as measured by a cuff on the right arm or directly by a catheter introduced through the mammary artery. If the pressure increases centrally, the pumping rate is increased. The aorta then may be clamped for significant periods and the aortic base of the ductus divided (*D*). The division is made so that maximum length is left for repair of the pulmonary end and a convenient field is provided for repair of the aortic defect (*E* and *F*).

Accidental tear of a ductus during repair can necessitate emergency cross-clamping of the aorta in the absence of preparations for hypothermia or systemic by-pass. Tapes are always placed about the aorta above and below the lesion at an early stage of the dissection to facilitate quick control, and suitable clamps are always at hand. Occlusion time adequate for secure repair is not likely to produce sequelae on the basis of the temporary ischemia, but the possibility of spinal cord damage exists. Cardiac strain is diminished by administering a sympathetic ganglion-blocking agent.

PLATE 80

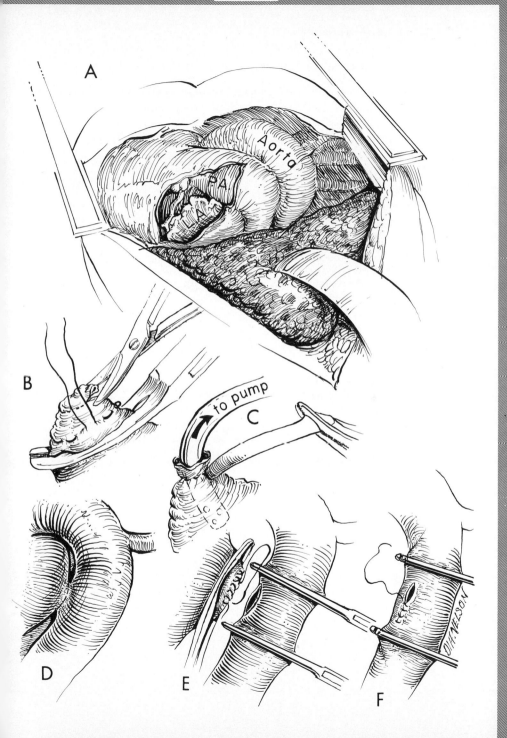

Repair by Excision and Direct Suture

The ease with which a coarctation of the aorta is repaired depends upon the anatomy of the deformity and the extensiveness of degenerative changes in the aorta around the lesion. The aim of surgery is to produce a broad anastomotic repair of the deformity so that no vestige of obstruction to circulation remains.

The patient is placed on his right side on the operating table, and left thoracotomy is done in relation to the fourth rib (*A*). The incision is posterolateral and through the bed of the fourth rib in adults. In young children less extension of the incision posteriorly is required, and the incision is made in the fourth intercostal space.

The first sign of pathology is seen as the soft tissues of the thoracic wall are incised and numerous large, thin-walled arterial collaterals are encountered. Blood loss during thoracotomy may be minimized by carrying the line of incision rather slowly through subcutaneous tissue and muscle, identifying and applying hemostats to these large vessels before they are cut. Otherwise a significant amount of blood will be lost unnecessarily.

Opening of the chest and retraction of the left lung downward and medially will reveal further evidences of development of collateral circulation. These include enlargement and tortuosity of the internal mammary artery and a marked enlargement of the left subclavian artery. Some of the intercostal vessels may be enlarged sufficiently to be visible under the parietal pleura adjacent to the upper descending aorta. A line of incision in the parietal pleura (*B*) is selected along the anterolateral aspect of the descending aorta and the lateral aspect of the subclavian artery.

[Repair of coarctation by excision and direct suture *continued on page 258.*]

PLATE 81

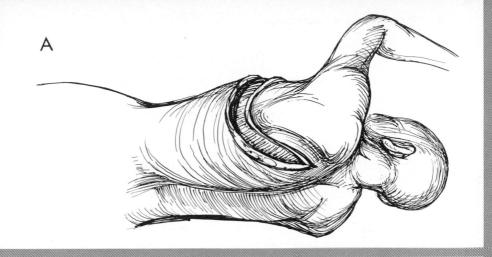

A

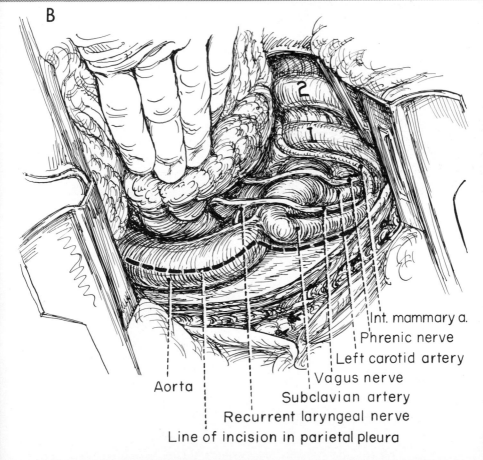

B

Int. mammary a.

Phrenic nerve

Left carotid artery

Aorta

Vagus nerve

Subclavian artery

Recurrent laryngeal nerve

Line of incision in parietal pleura

Sharp dissection is then continued along the wall of the aorta and subclavian artery (C). The stretching trauma of blunt dissection with a hemostat or scissors is avoided, particularly on the posterior surface of the aorta in relation to the large intercostal arteries. The end point of the dissection after ligation of the ligamentum arteriosum is shown in D. The aorta and subclavian artery are freely mobile. They are lifted up at the point of coarctation and for considerable distance above and below. Three to five intercostal artery pairs should be dissected to sufficient length that the mobilization of the distal aorta will be adequate for repair after resecting the constricted portion of the vessel.

It is noticed that the external appearance of constriction of the aorta is not as great as the high degree of obstruction would indicate. The local thickening of the aortic wall (E) accounts for this discrepancy. Clamps are placed above and below the area of coarctation, which is removed by clean incisions (F). The ends are trimmed so that the resulting lumens above and below are equal. In the rather common situation illustrated, it has been necessary to include a small portion of the proximal subclavian artery in the upper line of incision to gain the proper size.

[Repair of coarctation by excision and direct suture *continued on page 260.*]

PLATE 81

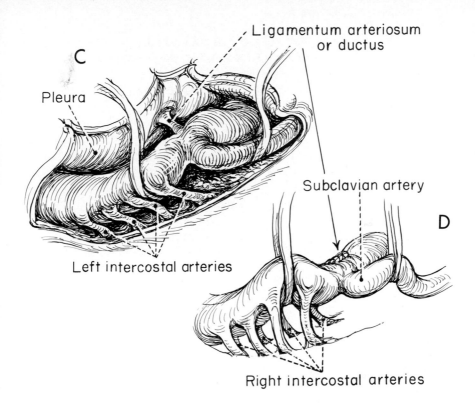

C

Pleura

Ligamentum arteriosum
or ductus

Left intercostal arteries

Subclavian artery

D

Right intercostal arteries

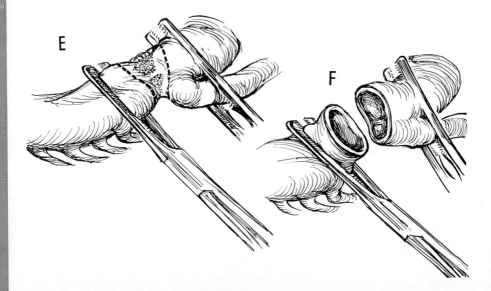

E

F

The anastomosis of the cut ends of aorta is carried out using any one of a variety of techniques. When there is great flexibility of the vessels, as in a very young person, placing of the posterior row of the anastomotic suture is facilitated by rotating the clamps to bring this row uppermost (*G* and *H*). However, the posterior row may equally well be placed without rotation of the clamps. The anterior row is introduced last (*I* and *J*). The distal clamp is removed first upon completion of the anastomosis, and any additional sutures required are put in before the proximal clamp is removed. Removal of the proximal clamp must be gradual. In order to prevent trauma to the vessel as it pulsates against the partially opened proximal clamp, finger compression of the aorta above the anastomosis may be substituted and the clamp removed from the field completely. The manual compression is then gradually relieved so that the heart will not suddenly be confronted with a marked change in peripheral resistance.

A double row of sutures may be used in the anastomosis, the internal layer being a continuous everting mattress suture and the external layer an over-and-over suture in the everted edges. The most commonly used anastomotic suture is illustrated in *K*. This is a simple over-and-over suture using fine arterial silk. The variations include a continuous everting mattress suture and interrupted sutures, either around the entire circumference of the anastomosis or on its anterior portion only. There is adequate evidence to support the view that interrupted sutures should be used when the coarctation resection is done in children under age 6, because continuous sutures of nonabsorbable material may interfere with growth in diameter of the line of anastomosis.

The repair is shown completed in *L*.

[Graft repair *on page 262*.]

PLATE 81

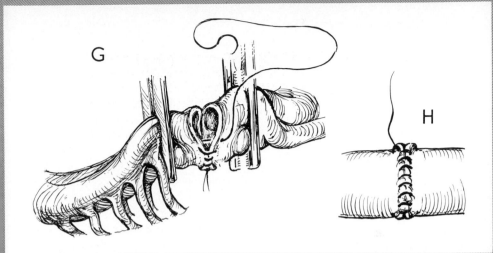

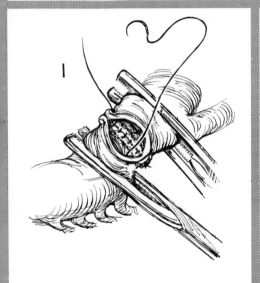

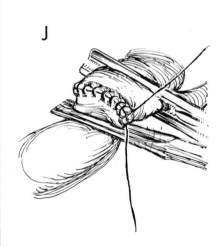

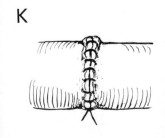

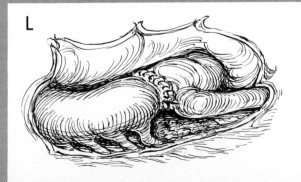

Resection and Graft Repair

A graft is found convenient to bridge the defect in the descending aorta after coarctation resection when there is marked loss of elasticity in the aorta. It is often necessary in older patients or when the coarctation is unusually long. Either a homologous aortic graft or a prosthesis is used.

A illustrates the completed dissection of a lesion in a 32-year-old patient in which the coarcted segment, measured between points of normal caliber above and below, was approximately 2 in. in length. The wall of the aorta in the region was deficient in elasticity and was fragile. The lesion was removed and a prosthesis selected. In *B* the proximal suture line to the prosthesis is completed. This anastomosis is conveniently done because of the mobility of the other end of the graft at this stage. A single layer, over-and-over suture line is used.

The graft is then pulled downward and cut at the point judged to provide proper length with moderate tension (*C*). The artery clamp is placed on the distal aorta beyond the first pair of intercostal arteries, and these vessels are clamped individually. This maneuver facilitates placement of the distal suture line because it frees a greater length of the distal aortic end. Since a maximum amount of vessel is not needed as in direct anastomosis, it does not matter that full advantage is not taken of the elasticity of this segment.

In constructing the distal suture line, the posterior row may be made from within the lumen after separate sutures are started from each half of the circumference. It is also possible to place each half of the suture from the usual position outside the vessel if the sutures are started at superior-inferior points bisecting the circumference. In this case a very small amount of rotation of the clamps suffices to bring the more remote side into view.

The relaxation of the vessels being anastomosed is probably more important in aortic suture than it is in any other situation. It is essential that the clamps counteract the elasticity of the artery and graft until the entire anastomosis is finished and ready to take this force as a unit (*D*).

PLATE 82

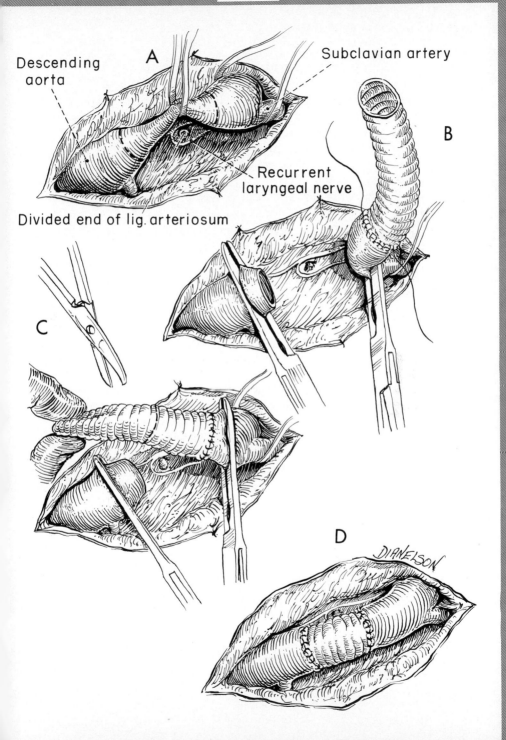

Descending aorta

A

Subclavian artery

B

Recurrent laryngeal nerve

Divided end of lig. arteriosum

C

D

DIANELSON

REPAIR OF COARCTATION PROXIMAL TO THE LEFT
SUBCLAVIAN ARTERY

Congenital constriction of the aorta sharply localized to the region between the left carotid and left subclavian arteries is one of several types of unusual coarctation of the thoracic aorta. Since the etiology of coarctation is not known, it is safe to say that this coarctation is related to the usual type only because of the identical nature of the pathologic anatomy. From a diagnostic standpoint, the fact that the blood pressure in the left arm is much reduced in comparison to that in the right is of little value because this is so often true in coarctations below the subclavian. The lesion may, therefore, be found unexpectedly at surgery.

On exposure of the chest cavity, the constricted appearance of the descending aorta at the usual site is not found. The left subclavian artery is large and the pulse in the descending aorta is diminished. The lesion is demonstrated after the distal arch has been exposed (*A*) through an incision in the parietal and mediastinal pleura. The vagus nerve is lifted on a cotton tape and its recurrent laryngeal branch is visualized passing in normal relation to a ligamentum arteriosum.

Ligation and division of the ligament (*B*) increases the mobility of the nerve structure and of the upper aorta. Secure ligation of the ligament is important since it may possess a small lumen.

Clamps are then applied to the thoroughly dissected aorta proximal and distal to the lesion (*C*), taking great care to avoid encroaching on the left common carotid artery. The force required to bring the cut ends of the aorta together for anastomosis is much less here than it is in coarctations of the usual type. The posterior suture row must, however, be placed from within the vessel, the anterior row of sutures being entirely accessible (*D*).

PLATE 83

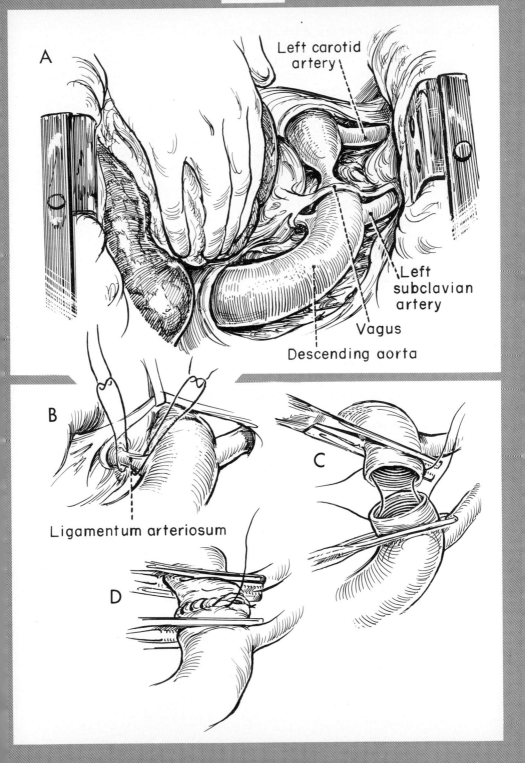

A

Left carotid artery

Left subclavian artery

Vagus

Descending aorta

B

Ligamentum arteriosum

C

D

Diagnosis of aorticopulmonary window is sometimes made at the time of a left thoracotomy for a supposed patent ductus arteriosus. It is probably best under these circumstances to discontinue the operation without carrying out any dissection in the region of the lesion. Fortunately, it is more usual that the diagnosis has been suggested by the clinical course of the patient and confirmed by aortography or catheterization.

Approach to the lesion is through a median sternotomy. Upon exposure (*A*), the great vessels at the base of the heart are found to be in their normal relationship, but the appearance is disturbed by the marked enlargement of the pulmonary artery. There is a gross thrill over the base of the pulmonary artery extending outward beyond its bifurcation. The aortic pulse pressure is palpably increased. The defect is in the adjacent walls of the aorta and pulmonary artery. It varies from 5 to 15 mm. in size, and its proximal edge may be as little as 5 mm. above the aortic valve ring. The semilunar valve annulus is normal on each side of the heart and the ventricular septum is intact. If the defect lies a maximum distance from the aortic valve ring, it is possible to isolate it and divide it between clamps. However, preparations must be at hand for institution of cardiopulmonary by-pass because isolation of the proximal edge of the defect may not be feasible without opening the pulmonary artery. *A* indicates the usual cannulations for by-pass, with the addition of a left atrial catheter.

After dissection is carried out around the lesion to the greatest extent possible (*B*), by-pass is started and the aorta and pulmonary artery are clamped distal to the communication. The pulmonary artery is opened (*C*), the incision being carried down to the defect and around it, leaving the aortic orifice intact for rapid closure. The aortic opening is closed without the necessity of applying a clamp at the defect. Immediately thereafter the clamp, which was placed distally, is removed to restore coronary blood flow. The pulmonary artery wall is redundant and any inaccuracies in the incision originally made around the defect can be compensated for during its repair (*D*). During the original dissection and during this period of closure of the pulmonary artery, the left coronary artery may be damaged, particularly if it has an unusually high origin, as illustrated here in figure *B*.

PLATE 84

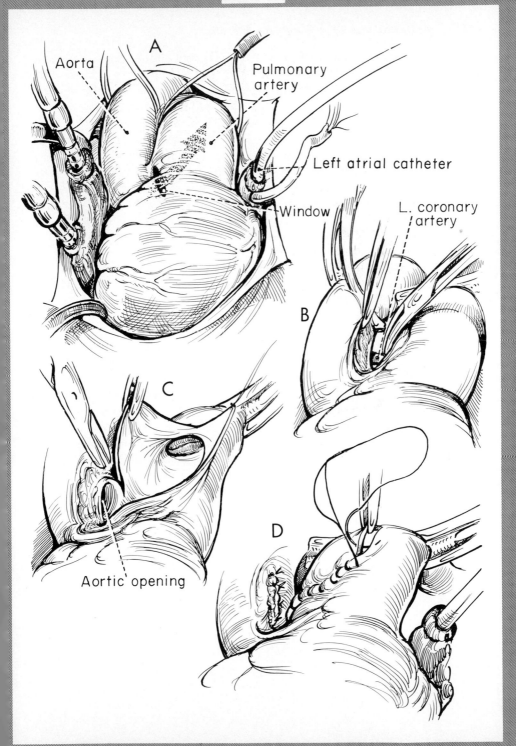

A — Aorta, Pulmonary artery, Left atrial catheter, Window

B — L. coronary artery

C — Aortic opening

D

The anomalous persistence of two aortic arches does not cause any vascular deficiencies in the brachiocephalic systems, but produces serious difficulties due to the compression of the trachea and esophagus which are enclosed within the ring formed by the double arch. Relief of the compression is obtained by surgical division of the ring at that point which will not disturb brachiocephalic circulation. Either the anterior or the posterior arch is small and, in order to maintain the flow through the arch, the smaller of the two is chosen for division.

DIVISION OF SMALLER ANTERIOR LIMB. — The form of the anomaly in which the anterior arch is small and the posterior arch of essentially normal size is diagrammed in *A*. In this anomaly the innominate artery usually arises from the ascending aorta at or just distal to the origin of the small anterior limb, while the left carotid artery arises from the anterior arch and the left subclavian artery arises either from the distal portion of the anterior arch or from the upper descending aorta beyond.

The surgical exposure obtained through a left anterolateral incision is shown in *B*. The vagus nerve, which lies anterior to all the vascular structures, is freed and elevated for its protection. It is evident that division of the anterior vessel at its point of entrance into the descending aorta would result in persistence of the tracheal compression because of the fixation of the anomalous arch by the left subclavian artery. Division between left subclavian and left carotid arteries will permit the carotid to fall forward because of its more medial fixation in the upper thorax. Division by ligation and transfixion suture as illustrated in *C* may be possible. However, if the space between the two vessels is small, the arch should be divided between atraumatic arterial clamps and the ends sutured in much the way a patent ductus arteriosus is managed (Plate 79). If the anterior arch and carotid artery continue to rest forcibly against the trachea, the vessels may be held away from the trachea by attaching them to the anterior chest wall, using fine sutures passed through the adventitia.

PLATE 85

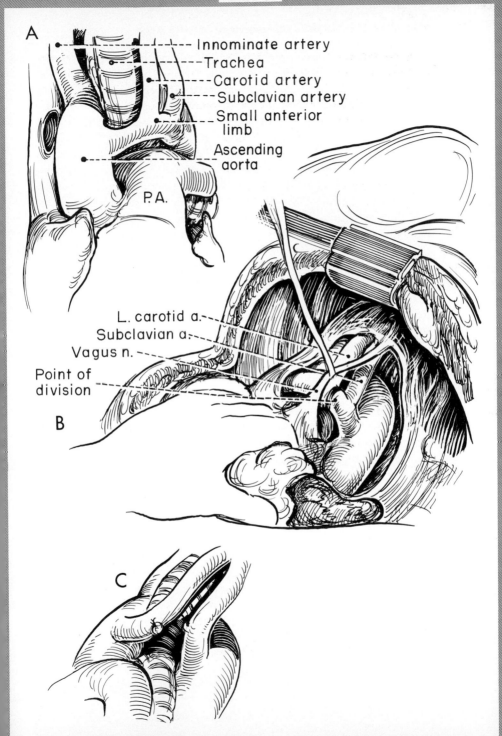

A

Innominate artery
Trachea
Carotid artery
Subclavian artery
Small anterior limb
Ascending aorta

P.A.

L. carotid a.
Subclavian a.
Vagus n.
Point of division

B

C

The variety of developmental anomalies of the aortic arch, the position of the ductus arteriosus and the origin of the brachiocephalic vessels strongly indicate the use of angiography to delineate the specific anomaly present in an individual case. Plate 86 illustrates two congenital malformations not related to duplication of the aortic arch.

CONSTRICTION OF MEDIASTINAL VISCERA BY LIGAMENTUM ARTERIOSUM IN RIGHT DESCENDING THORACIC AORTA. — An angiogram of the aortic arch in the anomaly diagrammed in *A* will show only the deviation of the descending thoracic aorta to the right. It will then be assumed that the relationship of the ligamentum arteriosum shown in the diagram exists and that its division will relieve the vascular ring.

The exposure in *B* is obtained through a left thoracotomy. Demonstration that one extremity of the constricting band is attached to the pulmonary artery identifies it conclusively as the ligamentum arteriosum. It is usually possible to ligate and divide this structure early in the procedure. This division improves the airway immediately, but it is important to continue the dissection between trachea and the vessels to ensure division of any fibrous bands that might maintain some degree of ring effect.

ANOMALOUS RIGHT SUBCLAVIAN ARTERY ORIGINATING FROM LEFT SIDE OF ARCH. — The anomalous right subclavian artery passes behind the trachea and esophagus in a diagonally upward direction, to leave the apex of the right chest in its normal location. This course is indicated in the diagram of the anomaly (*C*). Careful radiologic examination of the barium-filled esophagus will often show a characteristic obliquely transverse depression in the posterior wall of the esophagus.

When this anomaly is exposed through a left thoracotomy incision, the origin of the right subclavian artery is found to be posterior and somewhat inferior to that of the left subclavian artery (*D*). If the aorta and left subclavian artery are freed from surrounding structures and displaced anteriorly, this vessel can be isolated over a distance adequate for its ligation and division. Before ligation is completed, the presence of the right carotid pulse should be determined during a period of provisional obstruction.

PLATE 86

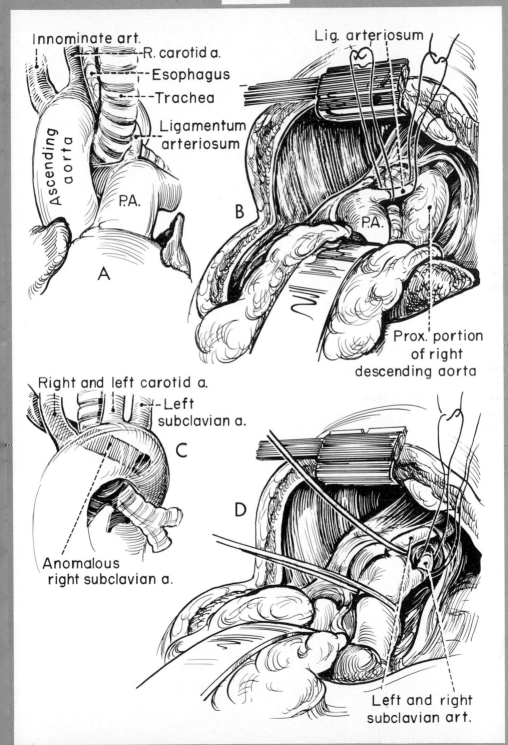

Innominate art.
R. carotid a.
Esophagus
Trachea
Ligamentum arteriosum
Ascending aorta
P.A.

A

Lig. arteriosum
P.A.
B
Prox. portion of right descending aorta

Right and left carotid a.
Left subclavian a.
C
Anomalous right subclavian a.

D
Left and right subclavian art.

CHAPTER 17

Pericardiectomy

CHANGES OCCURRING in the pericardium due to inflammatory disease may so restrict cardiac activity as to necessitate removal of the pericardial sac. These changes ordinarily are the late sequelae of an acute pericarditis and consist of the formation of an extensive scar involving the pericardium and epicardium. Less frequently, cardiac action may be inhibited by the edema and exudate accompanying the acute phase of the pericarditis. This situation, which occurs notably only in relation to a tuberculous infection, can require early pericardiectomy for removal of the diseased tissue and improvement of cardiac function. Healed tuberculosis is also a common etiology of constrictive pericarditis in which fibrosis and scar tissue formation are responsible for the effect on the heart. In many cases the etiology is indefinite and at the time the condition is seen, even if tuberculosis was the cause, it may no longer be identifiable pathologically. A history of the acute phase of pericarditis may not be elicited, and onset is at times very insidious. In chronic constrictive pericarditis the pericardium may be thick and densely adherent, and some degree of calcification is found in approximately 60 per cent of cases.

The clinical features of constrictive pericarditis depend on the extent of the disease and the amount of restriction of the heart brought about by the diminution in size of the pericardial sac that accompanies the fibrosis. This factor of restriction is more important than the fusion of epicardium to pericardium. All degrees of such fusion are seen, and in some the adhesions between these two layers are not prominent. Early complaints are shortness of breath on exertion and dependent edema. Later, enlargement of the liver, ascites and ankle edema become prominent. The heart is usually normal in size or only slightly enlarged. Increased venous pressure is evidenced in both the upper and lower extremities. The lesion does not produce murmurs and the heart sounds themselves are usually quiet. Fluoroscopic examination of the heart will disclose decreased pulsation, and the chest x-ray may show a layer of calcification on the surface of the cardiac shadow. A third heart sound, which is fairly often present, probably represents the heart's suddenly meeting the resistance of the pericardium during diastolic filling. The common electrocardiographic change is diminished voltage and flattening of the T waves. Direct measurement of the venous pressure in the right atrium is valuable, and cardiac catheterization shows a characteristic abnormality of the pressure curve in the right ventricle.

The results of surgery for chronic constrictive pericarditis are most gratifying. They depend, however, on the completeness with which the pericardiectomy is done. In the past, much emphasis was placed on the effects of constriction about the pericardial openings through which the venae cavae entered the heart. Although these structures are, indeed, encircled by the fibrotic process, the most important aspect of the physiologic effects is the restriction of the diastolic filling of the ventricles, not the impedance to flow of blood into the heart during diastole. Of the several approaches used, any which permits removal of as much of the thickened pericardium as possible is appropriate. The incisions vary from a small anterior left thoracotomy to an extensive bilateral trans-sternal thoracotomy. The midline vertical sternum-splitting incision has also been used. One of the thoracotomies which provides effective exposure for removal of the pericardial layer from both sides of the heart is described in Plate 87. It consists of a left thoracotomy through the fifth intercostal space, extended medially to transect the sternum and then into the fifth right intercostal space for a short distance. This approach affords good exposure of the ventricular bodies, both anteriorly and on the diaphragmatic surface. The pericardium over the right atrium may be removed as well as that in the area of the inferior vena cava.

Of the various incisions available for exposure, one which gives good access to all areas is a modified bilateral thoracotomy. The incision is in the left fifth intercostal space, extending from the posterior angle of the ribs anteriorly to and across the sternum (*A*). The fifth right intercostal space is also opened in continuity for a variable distance which may be as far as the midclavicular line. As shown in *A*, the skin incision on the left side does not necessarily extend posteriorly beyond the angle of the scapula. The intercostal incision, however, is carried beyond the skin incision as needed to gain mobility of the ribs for their retraction.

The left pleural cavity is opened and the lung retracted laterally (*B*). The right pleura is dissected from the pericardium and is left intact unless inseparable adhesions to the pericardium make this impractical. The site of initial incision through the pericardium must be selected blindly because of the thickness of the layer. It is best placed over the left ventricle, far enough to the left and posterior to avoid the general location of the anterior descending coronary artery.

This incision may uncover a plane between epicardium and pericardium in which the adhesions between the two layers are not of mature scar tissue. If this is so, the dissection between the two is carried out as the initial incision is lengthened and large areas of myocardium may be exposed rather quickly. If the adhesions are densely fibrous, the site tried initially may be abandoned for the time and another tried, or the incision simply carried down to that level at which motion signals the nearness of myocardium and the sharp dissection carried on laterally (*C*). If the two layers are easily separable, removal of the epicardium may not be necessary. The extent to which free expansion and contraction of the ventricles occurs after removal of the pericardium determines this point.

[Pericardiectomy *continued on page 276.*]

PLATE 87

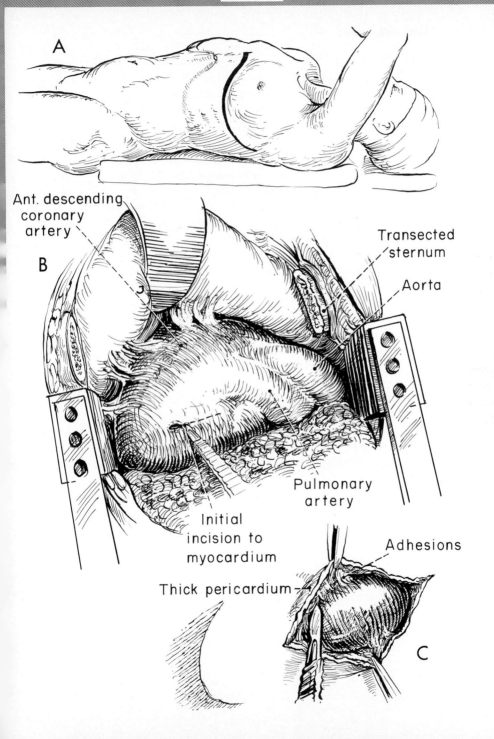

A

B

Ant. descending
coronary
artery

Transected
sternum

Aorta

Initial
incision to
myocardium

Pulmonary
artery

Thick pericardium

Adhesions

C

The requirements for pericardiectomy are met only when the operation has been done in a total fashion. Difficult areas are encountered usually along the atrioventricular groove on the left side where the coronary sinus and circumflex coronary artery must be protected and along the course of the anterior descending branch of the left coronary artery. All dissection is done with sharp instruments rather than with a spreading movement using scissors or a hemostat, because the latter motion may tear the structures which it is important to preserve (*D*).

The left phrenic nerve is exposed to danger principally while the specimen of thick pericardium is trimmed away as parts of it are freed. The nerve should be isolated early in the procedure and protected. If it is embedded in scar, a strip of the pericardium may easily be left in its course after being freed from the surface of the heart.

In *E*, the last stages of the dissection along the posterior aspect of the right ventricle and about the inferior vena cava are shown. By this time the heart has become relatively mobile. Its contractions are freer, and it is usually larger due to the release of the constriction. It can, therefore, be lifted out of the pericardial sac as the latter is dissected from the surface of the myocardium. The greatest danger of entry into a cardiac chamber exists during the dissection over the right ventricle. When such an incident occurs, it has been found convenient to provide hemostasis by finger pressure over the small perforation and to approach the region from other points around the periphery of the damaged area. It is well to leave some of the pericardium in the area adjacent to the tear or incision and to use this tougher material in its repair. An isolated small area of pericardium will not, in remaining, affect the mechanical relief of the constriction.

PLATE 87

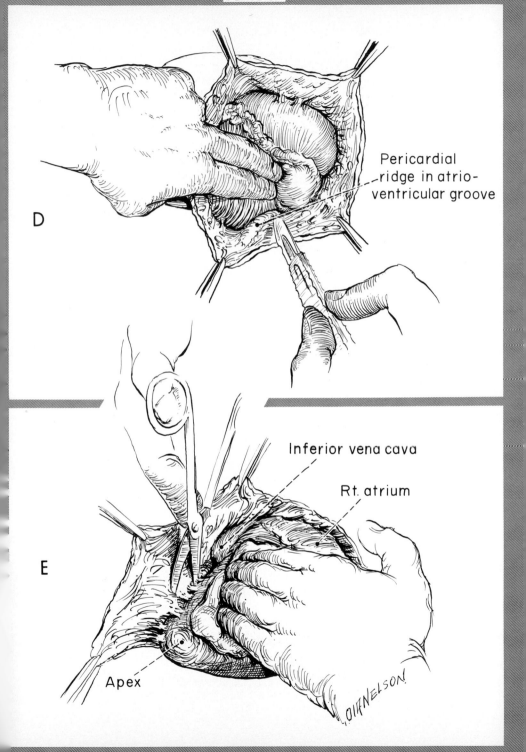

D

Pericardial ridge in atrio-ventricular groove

E

Inferior vena cava

Rt. atrium

Apex

CHAPTER **18**

Mitral Valve Surgery

Closed Mitral Commissurotomy

MANY YEARS' experience has led to the conclusion that closed mitral commissurotomy is a dependable treatment of choice for patients with isolated, noncalcific mitral stenosis without regurgitation or calcification.

The patient is placed on the operating table with the left side moderately elevated (*A*). The left arm is supported anteriorly and the hips are positioned in such a way as to render accessible both groin areas. This is done so that, in the event the closed-heart procedure must be converted to an open-heart operation because of the operative findings, an incision can be made in the groin (*B*) for heart-lung machine cannulation.

A fifth intercostal space anterolateral thoracotomy is used. The lung is retracted and the pericardium opened anterior to the phrenic nerve (*C*). The heart is examined and the left atrial appendage inspected for thrombus or evidence of systolic expansion indicating the presence of mitral insufficiency. If the atrial appendage is found to be thrombosed, the procedure should in most cases be converted to an open one with the pump-oxygenator. In exceptional circumstances the condition of the patient may warrant attempts to extract the thrombus from the appendage to provide a clot-free approach to the valve. If the appendage is free of clot, then a pursestring of heavy silk is placed at its base and a second, Teflon-pledget supported pursestring is placed at the thin area at the tip of the left ventricle (*D*). The appendage of the left atrium is then opened (*E*) and the orifice supported by two fine sutures of silk (*F*).

[Closed mitral commissurotomy *continued on page 280.*]

PLATE 88

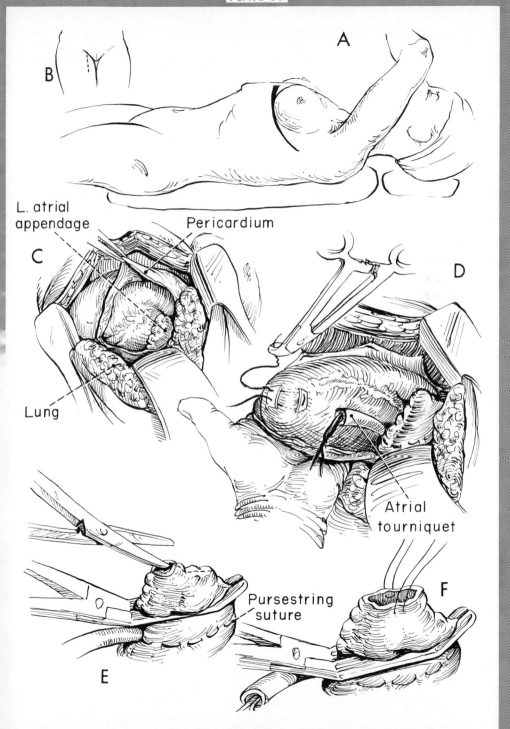

A

B

C L. atrial appendage   Pericardium

Lung

D

Atrial tourniquet

E

Pursestring suture

F

The index finger is then inserted through the atrial appendage and the character of the mitral valve noted. The severity of the stenosis, the presence or absence of mitral insufficiency, the mobility of the valve leaflets and the presence or absence of calcification are determined (*G*). An attempt is made to mobilize the fused commissures by application of lateral pressure from the exploring finger, and some increase in the valve orifice size is usually achieved. Most often, however, the opening remains unsatisfactory and instrumental fracture of the valve is done.

The transventricular dilator is passed retrograde through a stab wound created in the center of the pursestring which was applied to the apex of the left ventricle (*H*). The tip of the instrument is then engaged in the valve orifice (*I*) with its position confirmed by the exploring finger in the atrium. With this finger evaluating the accomplishment, the dilator opens the valve in small increments until a 3–4 cm. opening has been achieved (*J*). *K* shows the completed commissurotomy. Prior to withdrawal of the finger from the atrium, the functional achievement is assessed with particular attention to whether or not insufficiency of the valve has resulted from the valvulotomy. The atrium and ventricle are then secured and the redundant atrial appendage amputated.

PLATE 88

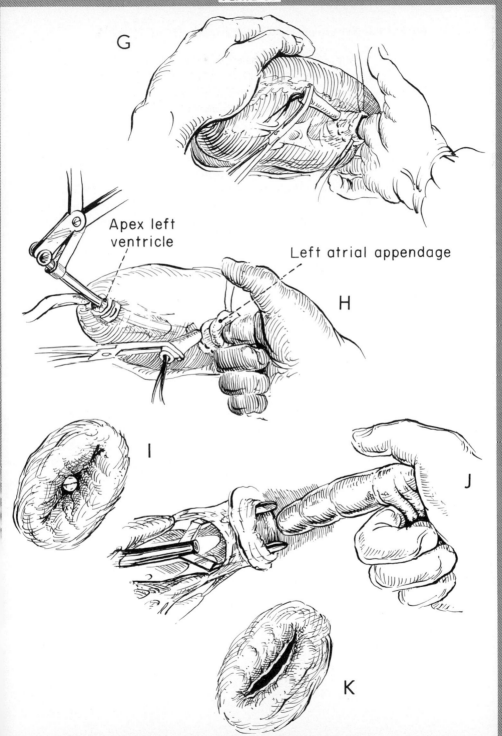

G

Apex left
ventricle

Left atrial appendage

H

I

J

K

Direct vision commissurotomy may be done either through the right or the left chest. Left-sided approach is seldom used, except when the open technique has been adopted because thrombi were found in the left atrium during a planned closed commissurotomy. With left thoracotomy, cannulation for the heart-lung machine is done using the femoral artery and vein; then, with partial cardio-pulmonary by-pass established, the heart can be retracted and a venous catheter placed in the right atrium.

Open mitral commissurotomy may be selected as a primary pro-cedure when the patient has previously had closed commissurotomy, when atrial clots are strongly suspected or when valvular replace-ment is a significant possibility.

A right fourth intercostal space anterolateral thoracotomy is cre-ated (A). Usually both the superior and inferior venae cavae are cannulated through the right atrial wall to provide for venous re-turn to the heart-lung machine. The superior and inferior venae cavae are then encircled with cord tapes or, alternately, the pulmo-nary artery is encircled to provide for venous occlusion during by-pass. After cardiopulmonary by-pass has been instituted, the heart is electrically fibrillated and the left atrium is opened posterior to the interatrial groove (B). After opening, the chamber is evacuated and then the interior is carefully inspected for thrombus. If a clot is present, it is meticulously removed, with particular care taken to prevent loss of fragments into the pulmonary veins. The mitral valve is then examined and the commissurotomy accomplished by incising or separating the valve leaflets between the two lines of attachment of the chordae tendineae (C). Subvalvular fusion of the chordae or even of papillary muscles may then be separated, as shown in D. A Crile dissector is useful in lifting the leaflets for examination or incision and also for separating subvalvular fusion. Pursestring ligation of the appendage may then be performed from inside the atrium to eliminate a nidus of potential thrombus for-mation.

PLATE 89

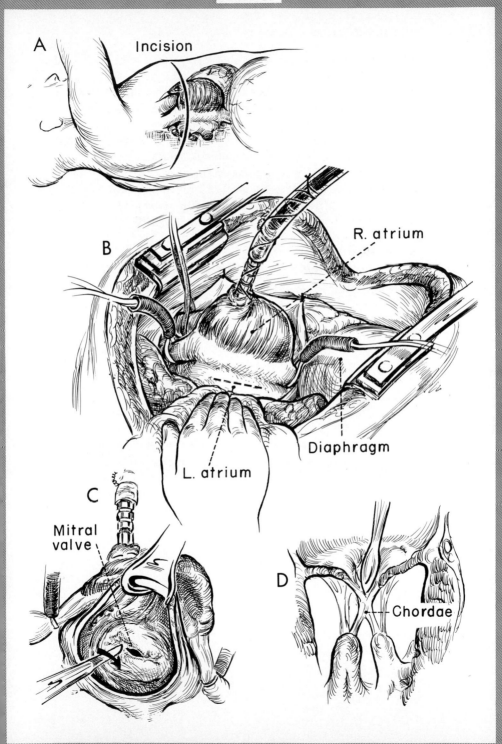

A

Incision

B

R. atrium

Diaphragm

L. atrium

C

Mitral
valve

D

Chordae

The surgeon must anticipate that valve replacement will be required in the vast majority of patients undergoing surgery for mitral insufficiency. Nevertheless, an occasional mitral valve can be made competent through a plastic repair. This is much to be preferred, as the consequences and long-term uncertainties of valve replacement can be avoided.

Plication of the mitral valve annulus at the extremity of each commissure is often the optimum procedure. Strong synthetic sutures are placed in a mattress pattern into the fibrous tissue of the annulus. These are passed through Teflon pledgets to prevent cutting through (*A*) and when tied, as shown in *B*, there is competence of the valve without excessive narrowing.

When there is severe loss of valve substance but yet a generous diameter to the annulus, it may occasionally be possible to mobilize and rotate one end of the larger leaflet, as illustrated in *C* through *E*, to achieve competency. Great care must be taken to avoid producing stenosis.

Free mitral regurgitation in the presence of a widely dilated annulus and torn chordae tendineae can sometimes be repaired by a similar maneuver without prior detachment of the leaflet. Such a transplantation, as shown in *F* and *G*, takes advantage of the fact that during ventricular systole the transplanted end of one leaflet is pressed against the underside of the other leaflet; thus, little stress is applied to the point of suture.

Accurate judgment is critical in making the decision to repair or to replace a valve. Whereas competency gained through repair is to be preferred, a plastic procedure may not achieve the goal of competency, the result being postoperative mortality or an unsatisfactory operation. Although there are disadvantages in valve replacement, competency and immediate improvement in hemodynamics can be assured.

PLATE 90

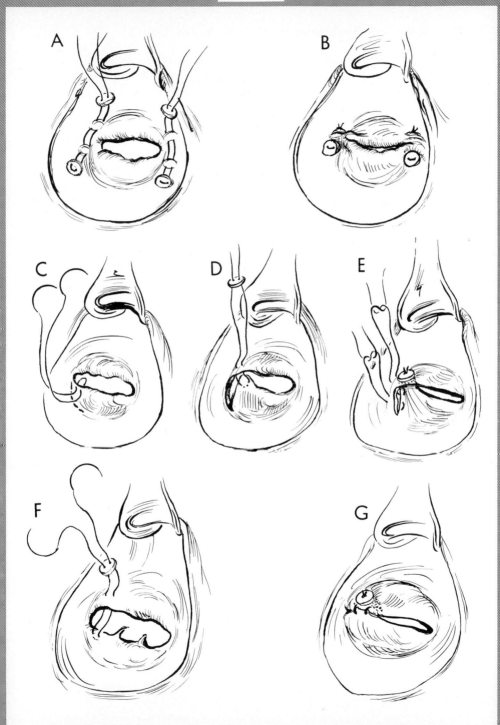

Most often, isolated mitral valve replacement is carried out through a right thoracotomy. Commonly, however, a median sternotomy incision is used (Plate 92), especially if the left atrium is large. The best exposure is achieved through a right chest incision, and less retraction of the heart is needed.

The patient is placed on the operating table with the right side moderately elevated, the right arm supported over the head and the groins positioned so as to be available for femoral artery and vein exposure (*A*). The fourth intercostal space is then entered, while the right femoral artery is exposed. After the pericardium is opened in front of the phrenic nerve and the superior and inferior venae cavae cannulated through the right atrium, cardiopulmonary by-pass is begun, using the femoral artery for arterial input to the patient. The heart is then electrically fibrillated and the venae cavae secured about the contained catheters. An alternate method obstructs the pulmonary artery instead; this forces blood from the coronary sinus out the caval catheters, rendering the left heart dry.

The atrium is opened posterior to the interatrial groove (*B*) and the chamber examined for thrombus. After careful removal of any encountered clot, the mitral valve is excised (*C*) with the underlying chordae and papillary muscles. Approximately 3 mm. of valve tissue is allowed to remain at the annulus to support the prosthetic valve sutures. If there is heavy calcification, especially if it extends below into the ventricular wall, it may be necessary to permit portions to remain. Miscalculation and overzealous removal of such deposits invading the annular rim or the adjacent myocardium may result in chamber perforation. Interrupted mattress sutures of 00 Teflon-coated Dacron are then placed in the mitral annulus (*D*). Suture depth is carefully judged to render the sutures secure but at the same time to avoid lateral injury to the aortic valve or the nearby coronary artery.

[Prosthetic replacement of mitral valve *continued on page 288*.]

PLATE 91

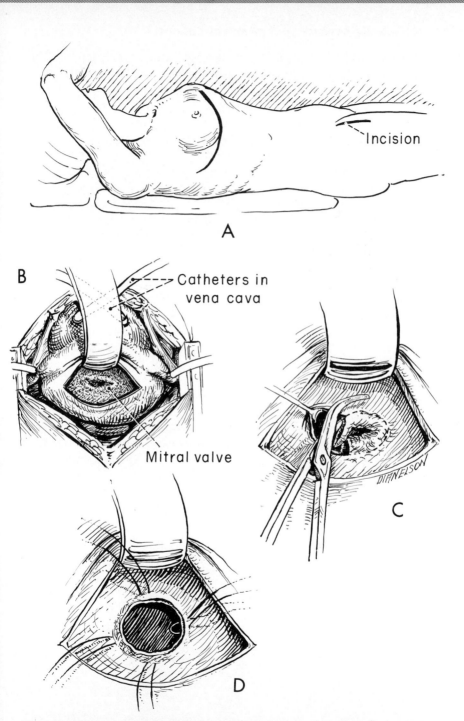

A

B

Catheters in
vena cava

Mitral valve

C

D

After all sutures are placed, they are fixed to the margin of the prosthesis (E) and the valve is then slid into position and the knots tied. A second pair of gloves is worn during the knot tying because of the tendency of the glove to tear with resultant contamination during this maneuver. As the knots are being tied, a Foley catheter is inserted into the valve and its balloon inflated to keep the valve incompetent (F). This is important to prevent the left ventricle from becoming a closed chamber as the mitral orifice becomes competent and then, with pressure distention of the ventricle, the aortic valve opening, possibly with the escape of trapped air into the aorta. The 16–20 sutures holding the valve are then cut. Purse-string encirclement of the appendage from within the atrium permits its exclusion and elimination as a focus of future thrombus formation.

The left atrium is then closed about the Foley catheter (G), allowing the heart to fill with blood as the suturing is completed. The uppermost part of the ascending aorta is then punctured with a large bore needle to create a vent for the escape of any air that passes from the heart into the aortic root. Firm inflation of the lungs by the anesthesiologist at this point will help expel any air from the pulmonary veins that has remained during atrial filling. The heart is then electrically defibrillated (H) and the catheter withdrawn from across the mitral valve. The left atrial closure is rendered secure by tightening a previously placed pursestring. During these maneuvers the vent in the aortic root is maintained to prevent air embolism.

PLATE 91

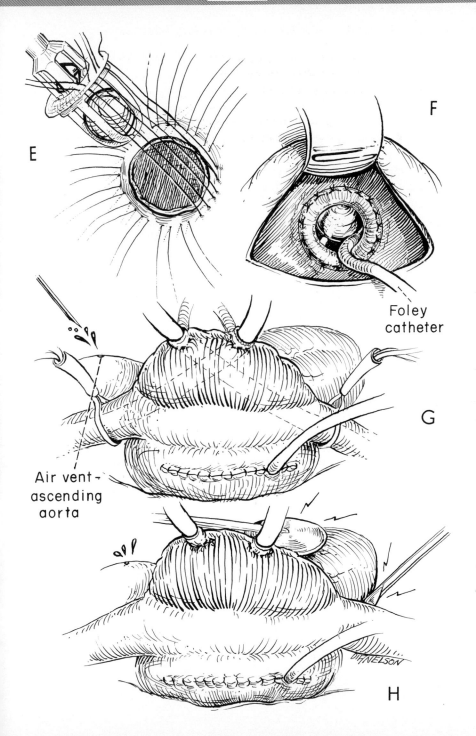

E

F

Foley
catheter

Air vent—
ascending
aorta

G

H

Mitral valve replacement may be readily done through a sternotomy when the left atrium enlargement is moderate to marked. Small atria give difficult exposure. Access to the aortic root and the desire to avoid opening the pleural spaces are additional reasons for using this approach. Because of the availability of the left ventricular apex for venting, maximum prevention of air embolism can be achieved.

After the incision (*A*) is made the pericardium is opened centrally, avoiding the pleural cavities. The superior and inferior venae cavae are intubated through the right atrium, and arterial input is provided through the femoral artery. With partial by-pass established, an apical vent is placed in the left ventricle. The pulmonary artery is then obstructed, the heart electrically fibrillated and the left atrium incised behind the interatrial groove (*B*). With retraction the mitral valve can be inspected (*C*) and then removed. During placement of the prosthesis, the valve is rendered incompetent with a Foley catheter (*D*). The left atrial appendage is ligated from within or without the left atrium to prevent a nidus of future clot formation. The atrium is then closed and the heart upturned so that the apical vent removes all air from the cardiac chambers. Expansion of the lungs by the anesthesiologist helps force any sequestrated air from the pulmonary veins. The heart is then defibrillated, the Foley catheter removed, the apical vent withdrawn and finally, cardiopulmonary by-pass discontinued and the venous catheters withdrawn (*E*). As in right thoracotomy mitral valve replacement, the uppermost portion of the ascending aorta is always punctured so that if there is escape of air into the aorta, it is vented to the outside without gaining access to the systemic circulation.

PLATE 92

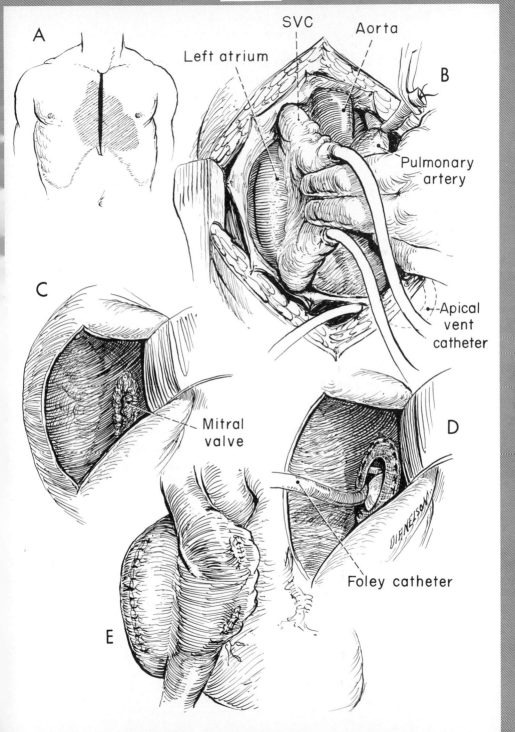

A

B

SVC

Aorta

Left atrium

Pulmonary artery

Apical vent catheter

C

Mitral valve

D

Foley catheter

E

DIBNELSON

CHAPTER 19

Aortic Valve Replacement

THE OPERATION is performed through a median sternotomy (*A*). The pericardium is incised in the midline and the remnant of thymus gland is divided between clamps and ligated, thereby giving maximum exposure to the heart and the ascending aorta (*B*). The distal ascending aorta is encircled and cord tapes are passed around the superior and inferior venae cavae (*C*). One of the femoral arteries is dissected and cannulated for arterial perfusion. The venae cavae are cannulated using the right atrial appendage and an area isolated with a pursestring suture over the right arterial wall (*C*). The patient is placed on total cardiopulmonary by-pass and the aorta is clamped proximal to the brachiocephalic artery. A sump catheter is inserted into the left ventricle through a stab wound at the cardiac apex (*D*). Either a transverse incision (*D*) or a longitudinal one (Plate 78) is then made in the aorta.

In the presence of a narrow aortic root, the use of transverse aortotomy should be avoided. Instead, a vertical incision in the right anterolateral aspect of the aorta extending into the noncoronary sinus of Valsalva should be utilized. Closure of this aortotomy with a generously wide elliptic patch of Teflon increases the clearance around the ball of the prosthesis and thereby helps prevent ascending aortic obstruction.

Once in the aorta, the coronary cannulas are introduced and myocardial oxygenation is maintained at normothermia. Certain precautions should be exercised to avoid coronary or myocardial injury. Careful placement of the catheter is particularly important in relation to the left coronary artery.

[Aortic valve replacement *continued on page 294.*]

PLATE 93

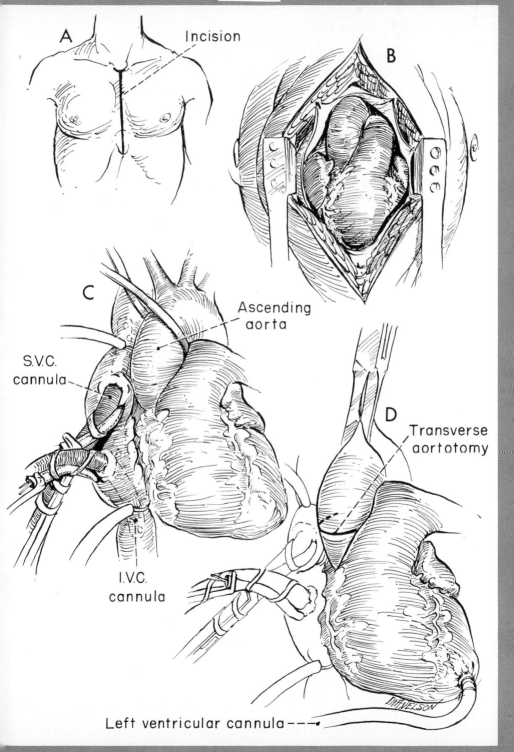

A Incision

B

C Ascending aorta

S.V.C. cannula

I.V.C. cannula

D Transverse aortotomy

Left ventricular cannula

Not infrequently the left coronary artery divides very close to its origin and, therefore, it is possible to pass the catheter blindly into one of the two main branche . Occasionally there are two adjacent orifices, one for the anterior descending artery and one for the circumflex branch. Under this circumstance it is best to introduce small catheters into both branches or to abandon left coronary perfusion if the duration of ischemia can be kept under 45 minutes. *E* shows the coronary catheters in place.

Excision of the aortic valve can prove tedious if it is massively calcified, with calcification invading the myocardium, the mitral valve or the aortic root. Thorough annular decalcification is done to permit proper placement of as large a prosthesis as possible. Care is taken not to dislodge any debris into the left ventricle or the left coronary artery.

An appropriate ball valve, determined by measurement of the annulus, is selected. Three transverse sutures previously placed at the base of each commissure are passed on either side of each strut through the sewing ring of the prosthesis (*F*). Three to five vertical mattress sutures are then placed in each division (*G*). The valve is lowered to the annulus, the operator making positively sure that the coronary ostia are not obstructed. Satisfactory maintenance of coronary perfusion assures the integrity of the coronary orifices and proper subcoronary placement of the prosthesis. The aortic incision is then closed, sometimes using two rows of sutures. The first is a continuous everting mattress suture and the second an over-and-over suture in the everted edges.

At this time, with the heart contracting, the left ventricular catheter is clamped, permitting the coronary flow returning from the lungs to displace air and fill the left heart chambers. The coronary catheters are removed as the aortic clamp is released, filling the ascending aorta and restoring retrograde coronary perfusion. The ventricular catheter attached to suction is now made functional to prevent ventricular distention.

In the presence of effective cardiac contractions, the left ventricular cannula is removed, the apex is repaired and the patient is taken off by-pass with gradual decrease in pump flow into the femoral artery.

PLATE 93

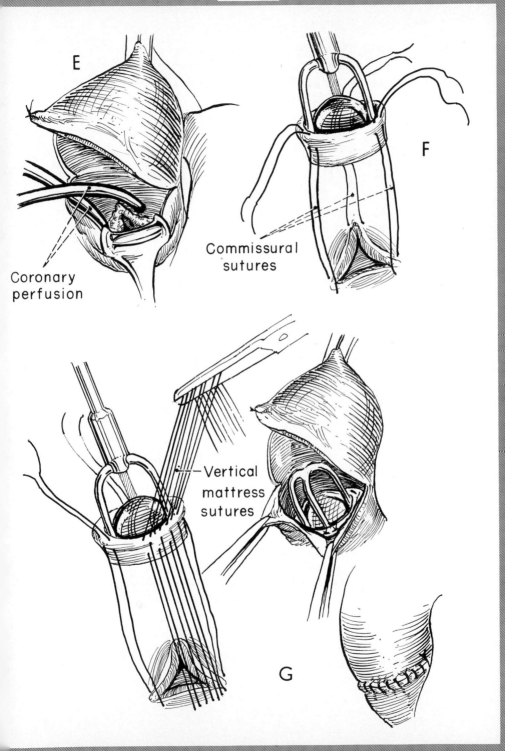

E

Coronary
perfusion

F

Commissural
sutures

Vertical
mattress
sutures

G

CHAPTER 20

Multiple Valve Operations

THE AORTIC AND MITRAL VALVES frequently are both damaged by rheumatic disease while the tricuspid valve is secondarily stretched and incompetent though much less often primarily diseased. Combinations of replacements, repair of regurgitation by various methods and commissurotomy, either open or closed, applied to combinations of aortic, mitral and tricuspid valves produce remarkable results in such cases. The most common double valve operation is mitral and aortic replacement, but a significant group of patients requiring aortic valve replacement have a stenotic mitral deformity which can be well managed by commissurotomy.

Tricuspid regurgitation is far more frequent than tricuspid stenosis as an indication for operating on this valve. Replacement or plication of the tricuspid valve is rarely required alone for acquired disease but either one is often added to an operation for mitral or mitral and aortic disease. Since the regurgitation is most frequently due to right heart dilatation, it is often reversible by intensified management before the mitral and aortic valve repair is done. Also, since the tricuspid regurgitation is so distinctly secondary to the load imposed on the right heart by a left-sided valve lesion, it might well recover after the repair of the latter. It is difficult to depend on this because the degree of overstretching of the tricuspid annulus may be beyond recovery. An attractive principle is that tricuspid incompetence which defies preoperative treatment be corrected at the same time as the left heart valves are repaired. This is in spite of the theoretically possible adverse effect of the suddenly imposed tricuspid competence on a right ventricle weakened by long-standing diastolic overfilling. The fact is that a heart subjected to mitral replacement recovers from the operation with difficulty if there is a significant residual tricuspid incompetence and this may be hazardous if the aortic valve was also repaired.

The decision as to which valves are to be repaired or replaced should be as definite as possible preoperatively on the basis of the physiologic and x-ray studies. This particularly applies to the incompetent aortic valve. Exploration of the two atrioventricular valves can readily be done and may yield the final evidence needed for a decision at the operating table. However, the same is not applicable to the aortic valve which is not conveniently palpated and is visualized only at the expense of an aortotomy. Even though aortic regurgitation is immediately evidenced when the cardiopulmonary by-pass is started, the leak is difficult to quantitate on the basis of the apparent rate of cardiac filling from the aorta.

The final decision as to which valves will actually be operated on must sometimes be made after physical exploration at the time of operation. In each such case there can be some question of the type of chest incision to be used. The mitral and tricuspid valves are more easily accessible through a right thoracotomy than a median sternotomy while the aortic valve is exposed from the right only with difficulty. The exposure from the right is improved by extension of the thoracotomy anteriorly across the sternum.

Multiple valve procedures including the aortic valve are generally done through the median sternotomy. In hearts requiring multiple procedures the atria are almost always significantly enlarged. They are both entered from the right cardiac aspect either through two atriotomies or through a right atriotomy and an incision in the interatrial septum.

When more than one valve is to be replaced by prostheses, the sequence is important. With the aorta clamped and opened and coronary perfusion instituted, the atrioventricular valve or valves are repaired first. This takes advantage of the great mobility of the heart which results from aortic cross-clamping combined with apical venting of the left ventricle.

Some of the major steps of a triple valve operation are outlined in Plate 94.

As shown in the inset, the median sternotomy incision is favored for procedures in which more than one valve is to be replaced. The guiding principle in this selection is the ease with which the aortic valve is approached and the coronary arteries are perfused.

After the institution of total cardiopulmonary by-pass, the ascending aorta is cross-clamped and the exposure to the aortic valve is provided by a longitudinal hockey-type incision or by a transverse supravalvular incision when there is significant aortic dilatation. The aortic valve is excised first. The calcium deposits are debrided carefully to avoid the loss of debris in the cavity of the left ventricle. Irrigation of the aortic root and the left ventricle with saline should follow to remove all particles. It has been our custom to use a Spencer catheter in the orifice of the left coronary artery and a Mayo tip in the right coronary ostia. In rare situations where the main left coronary artery is nonexistent or quite short, the anterior descending and circumflex branches should be cannulated separately. A perfusion flow rate which produces a pressure of about 60–80 mm. Hg has been found quite satisfactory. The heart often contracts rhythmically throughout the procedure.

The mitral valve is then exposed through a longitudinal incision behind the interatrial groove. The valve is totally excised and replaced with a proper size Starr-Edwards prosthesis. A continuous suture technique is preferred whenever possible. The left atrial incision is then repaired in two layers, leaving a small Foley catheter for maintaining incompetence of the mitral valve and removal of air from the left atrium at the end of the procedure.

The aortic valve is then replaced and the aortic incision closed securely after removal of air from the left side of the heart.

The tricuspid valve is exposed through a longitudinal incision anterior to the interatrial groove. A common alternative is the replacement of the tricuspid valve as the second step prior to aortic valve replacement.

Points of major importance are the maintenance of adequate coronary perfusion and rhythmic contractions of the heart. Thorough evacuation of residual air is imperative. This can be accomplished through the left ventricular vent and the aortic incision.

PLATE 94

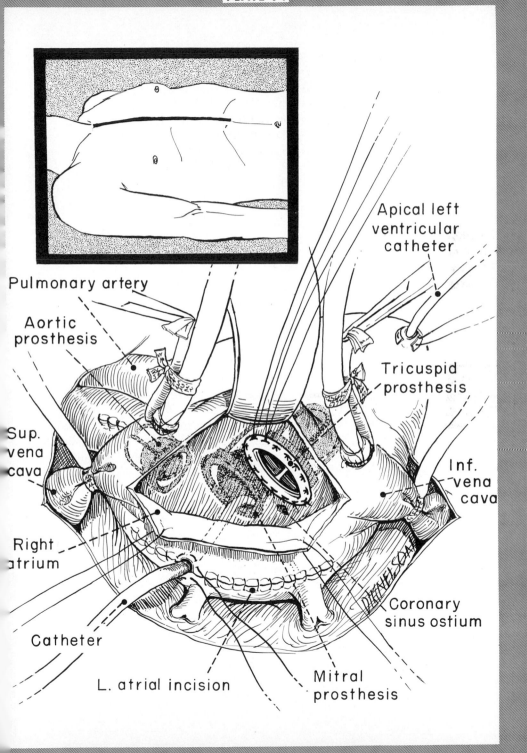

Apical left
ventricular
catheter

Pulmonary artery

Aortic
prosthesis

Tricuspid
prosthesis

Sup.
vena
cava

Inf.
vena
cava

Right
atrium

Coronary
sinus ostium

Catheter

L. atrial incision

Mitral
prosthesis

CHAPTER 21

Interatrial Septal Defects

Atrial Septal Defect

ATRIAL SEPTAL DEFECT is a common lesion among pa-
tients with congenital heart disease who reach adult age. Individuals
with uncomplicated atrial septal defect are often asymptomatic. Ex-
ertional dyspnea may be experienced if the left-to-right shunt is massive. Pulmonary resistance is normal in the initial stage, permitting
a huge shunt across the septal defect. Pulmonary vascular resistance gradually rises and the right-sided chambers enlarge. On rare
occasions pulmonary pressure rises above the systemic level, causing a reversal of shunt across the defect.

The diagnosis of atrial septal defect may be suspected in the
presence of a hyperdynamic and enlarged heart associated with
increased vascularity of the lungs, ejection systolic murmur over
the pulmonary artery, a fixed, widely split second sound and electrocardiographic evidence of right bundle branch block. A diastolic
rumble over the tricuspid valve is indicative of massive left-to-right
shunt, and a pansystolic murmur at the apex in addition to those
described above suggests a cleft atrioventricular valve.

The three common types of atrial septal defects are:

1. Ostium secundum—an elliptic defect at the fossa ovalis not
associated with other anomalies.

2. Sinus venosus—a defect situated high in the septum near the
orifice of the superior vena cava, often associated with partial anomalous connection of the right pulmonary veins.

3. Ostium primum—a round defect occurring low in the septum,
often associated with significant malformations of the atrioventricular valves.

PLATE 95

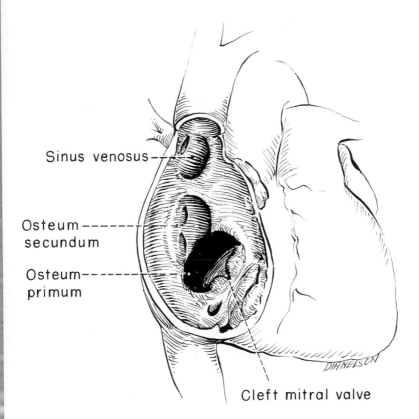

Sinus venosus

Osteum
secundum

Osteum
primum

Cleft mitral valve

Closure of the defect in asymptomatic infants with a left-to-right shunt of greater than 2:1 may be postponed to be performed electively before the child starts school. The operation is recommended even in older individuals with pulmonary hypertension, as long as a predominant left-to-right shunt still exists. Systemic pulmonary hypertension with a balanced shunt or a reversed shunt is a contraindication to surgical intervention.

The closure of the defect can be accomplished through a midsternotomy incision as well as through a right anterolateral fourth intercostal space incision. Cardiopulmonary by-pass is instituted, using the right atrial appendage for cannulation of the superior vena cava. The inferior vena cava catheter is introduced through a stab wound on the lateral wall of the right atrium and is secured in place with a pursestring suture. The arterial line is introduced through the femoral artery. Total by-pass is accomplished by constriction of the superior and inferior venae cavae with encircling cord tapes, using rubber tourniquets. To avoid air embolization, the aorta must be cross-clamped before the atrial incision is made or ventricular fibrillation must be induced electrically.

Ostium secundum can be exposed well through a transverse atriotomy (*A*). Placement of sutures at each end of the defect facilitates closure (*B*). A carefully placed single row of continuous suture will often suffice (*C*). Before completion of this suture line, air is evacuated from the left atrium by inflation of the lungs to fill the left atrium with blood returning from the lungs. The right atrium is then repaired, with particular attention to evacuation of air from the right atrium. The use of an aortic clamp is optional and provides a dry operative field.

Prior to termination of induced fibrillation, a puncture hole is made with a large needle in the ascending aorta to evacuate the residual air bubbles (*D*). Often sinus rhythm is resumed as soon as electrical fibrillation is terminated. Otherwise, the heart is defibrillated with a countershock and placed on a partial by-pass.

Termination of cardiopulmonary by-pass, neutralization of heparin and chest closure are done in the usual manner.

PLATE 96

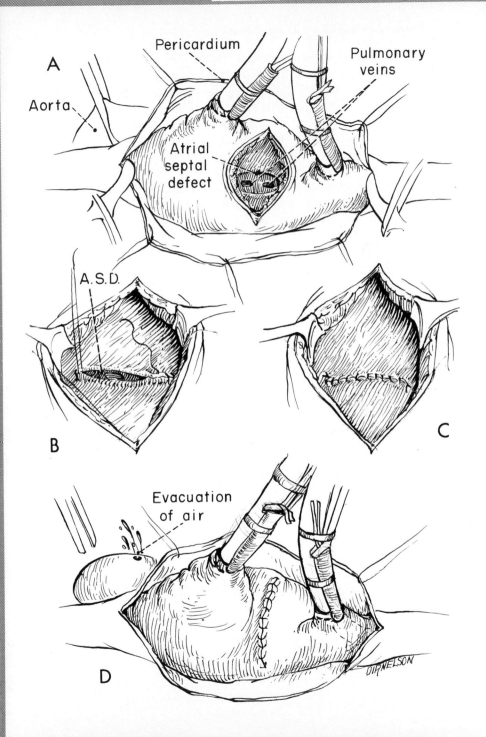

A
Aorta
Pericardium
Pulmonary veins
Atrial septal defect

B
A.S.D.

C

D
Evacuation of air

DITNELSON

The association of anomalous right lung drainage into the right atrium can only be recognized by cardiac catheterization and angiocardiography. The right upper lobe vein may enter the superior vena cava, presenting a challenging technical problem in regard to cannulation of the superior vena cava and repair of the defect. A careful dissection of the superior vena cava and the anomalous pulmonary vein is an important step prior to initiation of cardiopulmonary by-pass.

Proper closure of the sinus venosus defect with rerouting of the pulmonary vein flow into the left atrium often requires a patch graft. The use of pericardium has proved most satisfactory. Direct closure of the septal defect may constrict the ostia of the superior vena cava or pulmonary veins, leading to serious complications.

A 45-degree lateral position is quite satisfactory (*A*) unless there exists a left superior vena cava, in which case a mid-sternotomy incision is preferred. The atrial incision should be longitudinal (*B*) to give good exposure of the defect (*C*). A patch of pericardium the size of the defect is sutured to the upper edge of the defect, the posterior wall of the vena cava, the lateral wall of the right atrium anterior to the ostium of the anomalous pulmonary vein and the inferior margin of the defect. Finally the suture line is completed anteriorly (*D*).

Precautions discussed previously are required to evacuate air from the cardiac chambers.

In defects involving the superior vena cava, the partitioning with a patch graft may cause obstruction to the venous return, requiring plastic procedures on the superior vena cava. Implantation of an oval-shaped piece of pericardium over the narrowed segment of the vena cava often corrects the anomaly.

PLATE 97

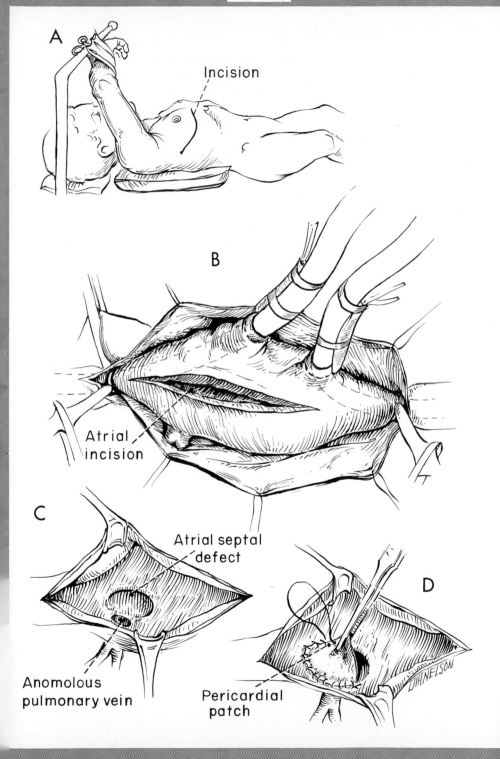

A

Incision

B

Atrial
incision

C

Atrial septal
defect

Anomolous
pulmonary vein

D

Pericardial
patch

The partial endocardial cushion defect known as ostium primum consists of a low-lying, large atrial septal defect associated commonly with a mitral cleft and occasionally with both mitral and tricuspid valve deformity. The presence of mitral or tricuspid regurgitation in a patient with clinical and physiologic findings of atrial septal defect indicate the likelihood of ostium primum. The life expectancy of patients with this lesion is definitely less than that of those with ostium secundum defect. Children may show evidence of congestive heart failure in infancy, urgently requiring surgical intervention.

The patient is placed in the supine position. A median sternotomy is the preferred approach. Cardiopulmonary by-pass is instituted, and the left ventricular vent is established through a stab wound at the apex. The aorta is cross-clamped intermittently to afford a dry field and a sluggish heartbeat. Exposure to the defect can best be obtained through a transverse atriotomy incision (*A*).

Closure of ostium primum defect should begin with repair of the cleft in the septal leaflet of the mitral valve (*B*). Several interrupted sutures placed from the annulus toward the free edge of the leaflet often correct the anomaly. Since the leaflet may be foreshortened, complete repair of the cleft may cause tenting of the leaflet and increased regurgitation.

A patch is always required for closure of the defect. Pericardium is preferred. Use of interrupted sutures (*C*) along the inferior margin of the defect away from the ostium of the coronary sinus avoids injury to the A-V bundle. The anterior and the superior edge of the defect may be repaired with a continuous suture. Evacuation of air remaining in the left atrium is accomplished prior to completion of the suture line.

The most serious technical complication is injury to the conduction system. If heart block occurs during operation, a temporary pacemaker wire should be sutured to the right ventricle and brought out through the skin below the anterior rib margin. The indifferent electrode can be implanted subcutaneously. If the heart block persists, a transvenous permanent pacemaker should be implanted before the patient is discharged from the hospital.

PLATE 98

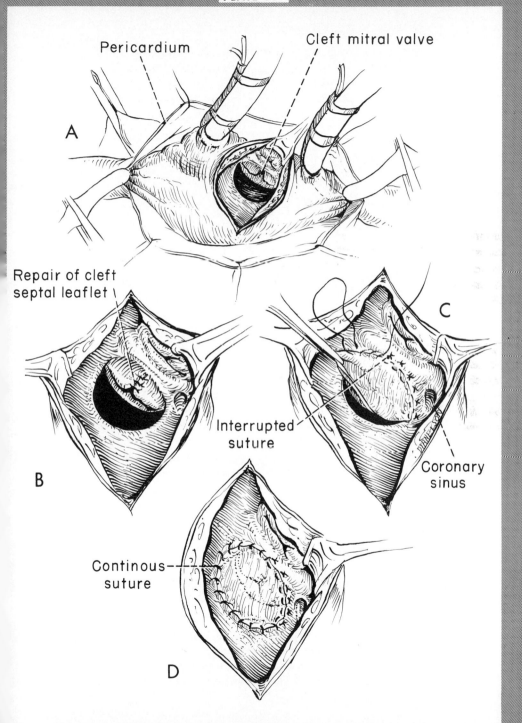

A — Pericardium — Cleft mitral valve

B — Repair of cleft septal leaflet — Interrupted suture

C — Interrupted suture — Coronary sinus

D — Continous suture

CHAPTER 22

Interventricular Septal Defects

VENTRICULAR SEPTAL DEFECTS occur in various anatomic locations. The functional disturbance depends on the size
of the defect. A small defect is compatible with normal life expectancy and may close spontaneously. Large defects allow large left-
to-right shunt and eventual equalization of the pressure in both
ventricles due to increased pulmonary vascular resistance. Once the
shunt becomes predominantly right to left, the lesion is inoperable.

Ventricular septal defects may be divided into outflow, inflow
and combined inflow and outflow defects (Plate 99). An uncommon lesion of left ventricular-right atrial communication can also
be included.

Inflow defects are found in the posterior muscular septum, often
beneath the septal cusp of the tricuspid valve beneath the aorta in
an area where the A-V conduction bundle traverses the postero-
inferior margin of the defect. Since this defect is posterior to the
crista supraventricularis, it may also involve the pars membranacea.

Outflow defects are situated between the crista supraventricularis and the pulmonary valve. They are comparatively uncommon.

Combined inflow and outflow defects are rare. They occupy a
large portion of the muscular septum.

Indications for primary repair of ventricular septal defect depend
on symptoms and the degree of left-to-right shunt. Children with a
small defect and normal pulmonary artery pressure do not require
operation unless there is a history of repeated subacute bacterial
endocarditis. Open-heart repair of ventricular septal defect should
be postponed, if at all possible, until the child is 4–5 years.

PLATE 99

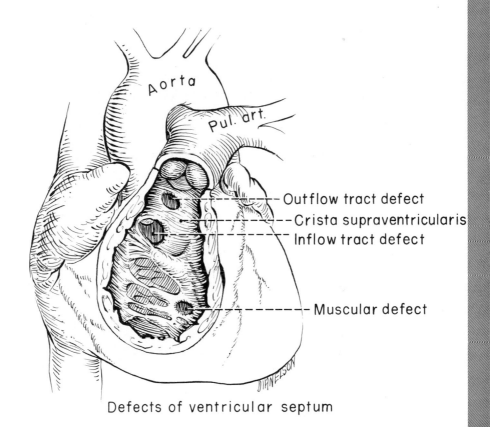

Aorta

Pul. art.

Outflow tract defect
Crista supraventricularis
Inflow tract defect

Muscular defect

Defects of ventricular septum

Repair is performed using cardiopulmonary by-pass, with the patient in the supine position. A median sternotomy (*A*) affords excellent exposure. Use of a left ventricular vent insures a dry operative field. A catheter connected to a metal tip is introduced through a stab wound at the apex of the left ventricle (*B*). This catheter is connected to the suction end and the blood is returned to the perfusion chamber. Total by-pass is accomplished by tightening caval tourniquets. The aorta is cross-clamped to allow muscle relaxation and to avoid air embolization.

Exposure of the ventricular septal defect of the pars membranacea type can best be obtained through a right atrial incision. This is particularly true when a left ventricular-right atrial shunt is present. The choice of primary closure of the defect or the use of a Dacron patch graft depends on the size of the defect and the quality of the margin. Other types of ventricular septal defects are exposed through a transverse incision in the outflow tract of the right ventricle (*B*). The septal leaflet of the tricuspid valve may cover the inflow type defects, requiring gentle retraction of the valve inferiorly to expose the lower margin (*C*).

The use of a Dacron patch for repair of ventricular septal defect is almost routine. Interrupted sutures should be placed superficially along the inferoposterior margin of the defect to avoid injury to the conduction system (*D*). All the interrupted sutures are placed first before tying them down in order to provide maximum exposure. The rest of the repair may be done with a continuous suture line (*E*). By introduction of the index finger into the pulmonary artery, the outflow tract of the right ventricle and the pulmonary valve may be evaluated. The repair of the ventriculotomy is then accomplished with two rows of suture. Air is allowed to escape through the left ventricular vent and needle holes are made on the anterior wall of the ascending aorta.

Resumption of coronary perfusion often results in return of sinus rhythm. Occasionally defibrillation is needed.

PLATE 100

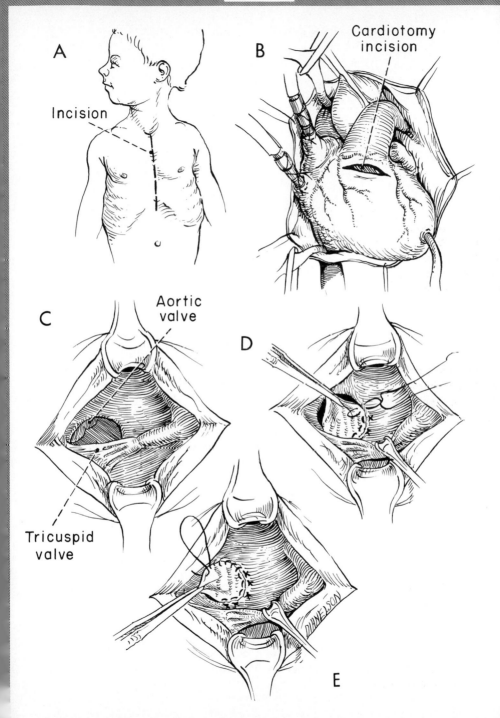

A — Incision

B — Cardiotomy incision

C — Aortic valve / Tricuspid valve

D

E

CHAPTER 23

Other Operations for Congenital Heart Defects

Palliative Surgery

INTRACARDIAC REPAIR of congenital heart defects is associated with high mortality in small infants. The appearance of congestive heart failure due to increased pulmonary flow nonresponsive to medical management, or of hypoxemic spells during infancy due to inadequate pulmonary flow, is an indication for operative intervention. The first palliative procedure devised to increase pulmonary circulation in patients with congenital cyanotic heart disease was developed by Blalock and Taussig in the mid-1940s. Since then various methods for systemic pulmonary shunt have been devised.

Intractable congestive failure due to increased pulmonary flow can be treated by pulmonary banding during early infancy. This procedure is applicable for patients with a large ventricular septal defect, with or without associated anomalies. Inadequate admixture of venous and arterial blood in complicated congenital defects such as transposition anomalies can be palliated by creation of an atrial septal defect or by increasing the size of the atrial septal defect, if present. This objective can often be accomplished by a balloon septostomy; if this is not successful, there is a strong indication for surgical enlargement of the atrial septal defect to increase the arterial oxygen saturation. In patients whose congenital anomaly permits intracardiac repair at a later date, the palliative procedure should be planned in a manner to allow easy accessibility for later repair.

Other palliative measures of tremendous benefit in this age group include division of patent ductus arteriosus in complex anomalies which result in congestive failure due to increased pulmonary flow, and superior vena cava-right pulmonary artery shunt, as developed by W. W. L. Glenn, in irreparable right-sided congenital lesions such as tricuspid or pulmonary atresia.

Ventricular septal defect is a common cardiac malformation in infancy and childhood. Most patients survive infancy. Many of these infants, however, cannot compensate for the increased pulmonary blood flow and congestive failure develops. Lack of favorable response to medical therapy indicates the need for surgical intervention. Pulmonary artery banding is used as a palliative measure in acutely ill infants.

The infant is placed in a 45-degree lateral position. Through a left fourth intercostal space incision the chest cavity is entered (*A*). The presence of a patent ductus arteriosus is determined first (the repair of patent ductus arteriosus is described in Chapter 16). The pericardium is then incised longitudinally anterior to the phrenic nerve (*B*). The pulmonary artery is carefully dissected free to permit passage of a narrow Teflon tape around the main pulmonary artery immediately above the pulmonary valve (*C*). The pulmonary artery is then constricted sufficiently to reduce distal pressure to about half its original value. The tape is secured in place with multiple mattress sutures (*D*). The pericardium is then partially closed.

Removal of a pulmonary band at a later stage may be difficult because of dense scarring. If the lumen of the pulmonary artery is not adequate at the time of intracardiac repair of ventricular septal defect, a longitudinal incision over the banded segment and repair of the vessel with an oval-shaped patch of pericardium corrects the constriction satisfactorily.

PLATE 101

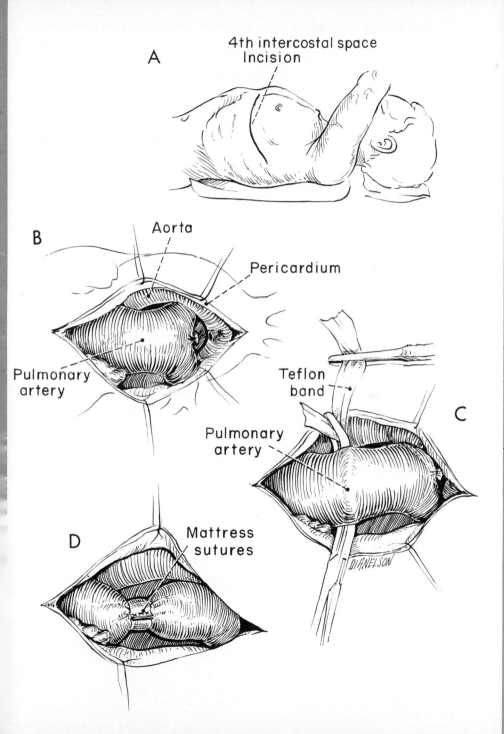

A
4th intercostal space
Incision

B
Aorta
Pericardium
Pulmonary
artery

C
Teflon
band
Pulmonary
artery

D
Mattress
sutures

DI.A.NELSON

This operative procedure should be reserved for infants with congenital cyanotic heart disease who have diminished pulmonary blood flow. In infants and children below the age of 5 years the side used is the one on which the subclavian artery arises from an innominate artery. A right aortic arch is usually accompanied by a left innominate and left thoracotomy is used. This is frequently the case in tetralogy of Fallot (*B*).

The patient is placed in a 45-degree lateral position, with the left arm suspended overhead (*A*). The goal of this procedure is to establish an anastomosis between the subclavian artery and the left pulmonary artery. Through a left-sided anterolateral fourth intercostal space thoracotomy, the thoracic cage is entered. The lung is retracted and the subclavian artery is dissected free as far laterally as possible. The vertebral branch and thyrocervical branch may be ligated (*C*). The subclavian artery is then transected and rotated downward to allow anastomosis between the end of this vessel and the side of the pulmonary artery. After adequate dissection of the pulmonary artery and proper proximal and distal cross-clamping, a longitudinal incision is made along the upper border of the pulmonary artery, and an end-to-side anastomosis is accomplished (*D*). The posterior edges are approximated first by a continuous row of fine synthetic sutures. *E* demonstrates the completed anastomosis and the direction of flow supplying increased blood to the ischemic lungs. The patency of the anastomosis can be confirmed by the presence of a thrill over the pulmonary artery. The chest wound is repaired in layers. A tube is left in the pleural space and is connected to a water-sealed drainage system.

PLATE 102

A

Incision

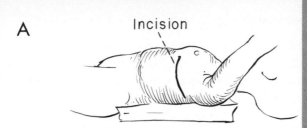

B

Right sided
aortic arch

C

Aorta

Pul. art.

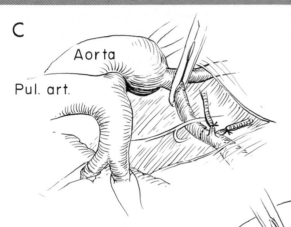

D

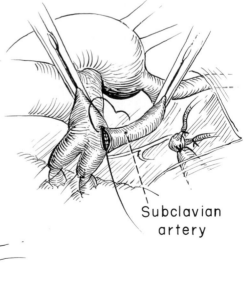

Subclavian
artery

E

Subclavian
pulmonary shunt

Transposition of the great vessels is the commonest cause of death from congenital heart disease during the first year of life. The technical difficulties and harmful effects of open-heart surgery at this early age underline the wisdom of palliative procedures to help these infants survive early infancy and to reach an optimum age for complete repair of the anomaly.

The fundamental cause of death in this defect is severe hypoxia. Oxygenated blood in the left side of the heart must gain access to the aorta which arises from the right ventricle. Admixture of blood between the two circuits takes place through communications such as patent ductus arteriosus and atrial and ventricular septal defects. The purpose of the operative intervention is to enlarge or create an atrial septal defect. This palliative procedure improves intracardiac mixing, it lowers the left atrial pressure and it prepares the atria for subsequent intracardiac repair.

The patient is placed in a 45-degree lateral position. A right submammary incision along the fifth intercostal space is made (*A*). The chest cavity is entered. The lung is retracted posteriorly and the pericardium is incised longitudinally posterior to the phrenic nerve. The right pulmonary veins and right pulmonary artery are dissected free and encircled with heavy silk ligatures (*B*). The pulmonary artery is clamped and the pulmonary vein ligatures are tightened to stop flow to and from the right lung. A vascular clamp of proper size is positioned with one blade along the anterior surface of the right atrium and the other blade along the posterior surface of the left atrium (*C*). Longitudinal incisions in the right and left atria on either side of the septum are made within the confines of the clamp. The septum is grasped with a clamp and gently withdrawn as the vascular clamp is temporarily loosened. As much of the atrial septum as possible is excised (*D*). The atrial incision is then repaired, approximating the edges of right and left atrial tissue (*E*). The clamp and ligatures are removed. Oxygen saturation of blood entering the aorta is thus increased by better mixing of atrial blood (*F*).

PLATE 103

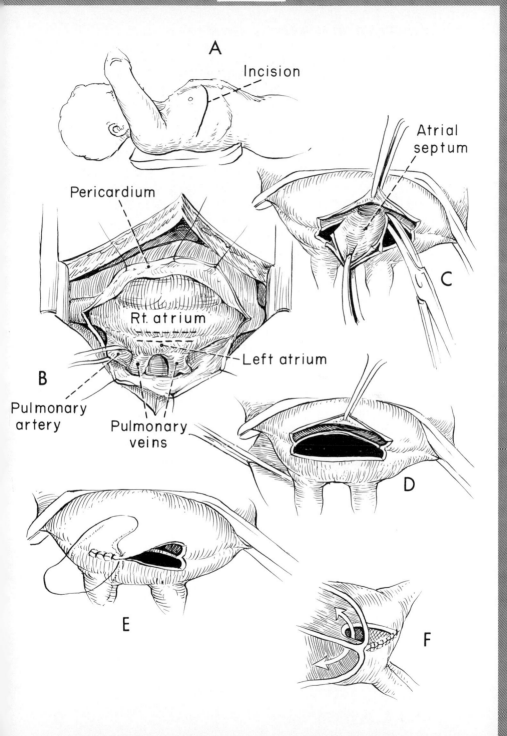

A

Incision

Atrial
septum

Pericardium

C

Rt. atrium

Left atrium

B

Pulmonary
artery

Pulmonary
veins

D

E

F

The major advantage of establishing a systemic pulmonary shunt using the intrapericardial portion of the aorta (A) is the ease of exposure and repair during the subsequent total intracardiac operation.

The patient is placed in a 45-degree anterolateral position. A right submammary incision is made extending from the right border of the sternum to the posterior axillary line. Through the fourth intercostal space, the chest cavity is entered (B). The lung is retracted posteriorly. The pericardium is incised longitudinally anterior to the phrenic nerve. The superior vena cava is dissected free from the right pulmonary artery and is retracted laterally. The right pulmonary artery is dissected free medial to its origin. A heavy silk suture is looped around the right pulmonary artery proximally to the left of the ascending aorta, and a control ligature of heavy silk is passed around the distal end of the right pulmonary artery (C). The control ligatures are tightened and a partially occluding vascular clamp is placed along the posterior aspect of the ascending aorta, excluding a portion of the aorta and completely occluding the proximal end of the right pulmonary artery (D). Five-millimeter incisions are made in adjacent portions of the aorta and pulmonary artery. These incisions are joined with a continuous suture of 6 – 0 synthetic material (E). Careful attention to the size of the anastomosis (F) reduces the incidence of postoperative congestive failure.

At the time of definitive surgery the ascending aorta-right pulmonary artery shunt can be repaired easily through a mid-sternotomy incision. After cardiopulmonary by-pass is established, the aorta is cross-clamped between the area of the shunt and the innominate origin. A longitudinal incision on the anterior wall of the aorta exposes the aortopulmonary anastomosis, permitting primary closure.

PLATE 104

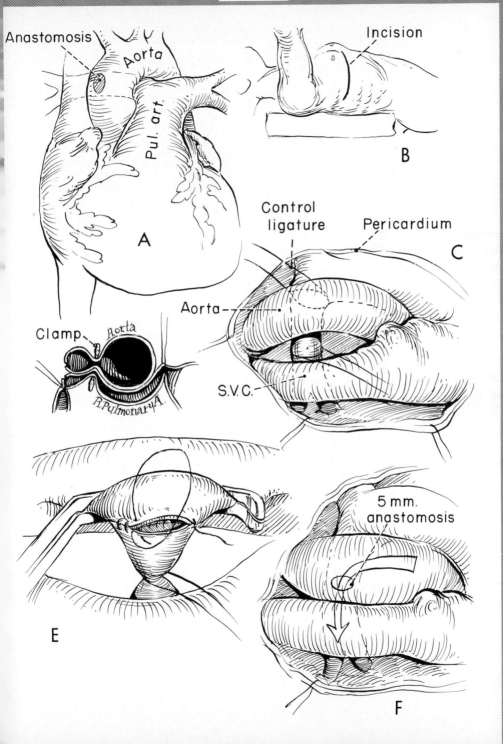

MUSTARD OPERATION

Since infants born with transposition of the great vessels rarely survive the first year of life, a palliative measure in early infancy is the first stage in preparation for total correction at a later date. Enlargement or creation of an atrial septal defect is most urgent in children who are deeply cyanotic at birth. This group of patients with transposition of the great vessels make the most ideal candidates for total correction because of their lack of accompanying intra- and extracardiac lesions. Atrial septal defects may be enlarged by a closed technique employing balloon-tipped catheters, or a Blalock-Hanlon procedure or a direct vision procedure using inflow occlusion may be done.

In the Mustard procedure a baffle of pericardium is sutured in place to reverse the venous inflow within the atrial cavity. The pulmonary venous return is directed into the right ventricle through the tricuspid valve, and the systemic venous return is channeled into the left ventricle through the mitral valve.

The approach is made through a median sternotomy incision. An oblong piece of pericardium 2 – 3 in. in diameter is excised, cleared of fat and soaked in heparin. The venous cannulations are established through right atrial incisions close to the caval junctions (*A*). The arterial line is introduced through the right common femoral artery. Total by-pass is instituted by tightening caval tourniquets. The ascending aorta is cross-clamped. A curved longitudinal incision is made in the wall of the right atrium close to the interatrial groove. Repair of ventricular septal defect, if present, can be accomplished by appropriate suture technique. Retraction of the septal leaflet of the tricuspid valve or detachment of the leaflet from the annulus may be necessary to expose the ventricular septal defect. The entire atrial septum is then excised (*C*), if necessary, going outside the heart superiorly to insure a large communication between the two atria. The defect created in the atrial wall is repaired by primary approximation of the cut edge.

[Correction of transposition of great vessels *continued on page 324.*]

PLATE 105

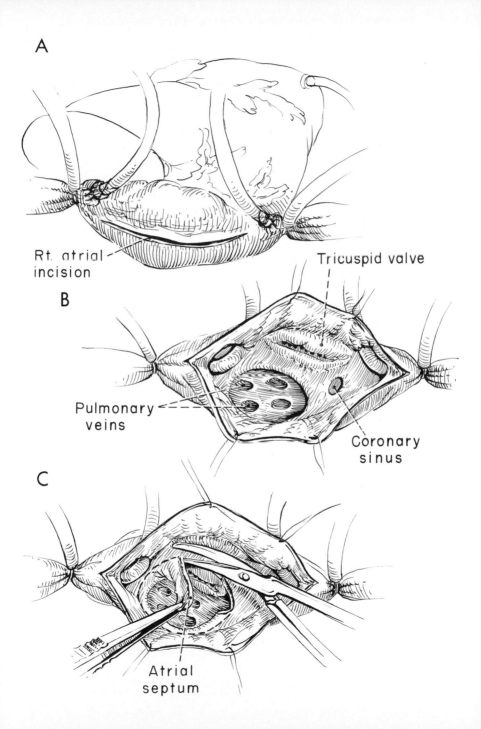

A

Rt. atrial
incision

B

Tricuspid valve

Pulmonary
veins

Coronary
sinus

C

Atrial
septum

To assure proper drainage of the coronary sinus blood into the newly created systemic atrium, the septum between the coronary vein and the atrium is cut with scissors (*D*). The pulmonary veins are identified and, with the use of a double-armed suture, the midpoint of the pericardial edge is fixed to the left atrium in the manner shown in *E*. The pericardial edge is then sutured in place around the entrance of pulmonary veins crossing the septum superiorly and inferiorly. The suture line then curves anteriorly over the catheters draining the superior and inferior venae cavae. The repair is completed by the approximation of the opposite edge of the pericardial patch with the anterior border of the atrial septum.

At the termination of the suture line the pulmonary veins enter the right atrium on the surgeon's side of the pericardial patch, and their flow is directed through the tricuspid valve into the aorta. The openings of the venae cavae and coronary sinus are hidden from view by the baffle and drain into the pulmonary artery through the mitral valve and left ventricle (*F*). The positioning of the pericardium within the atria should be accomplished in such a manner that the baffle divides the atria evenly and allows adequate capacity in each atrium. If necessary, it is possible to enlarge the capacity of the right atrium by using a pericardial patch in closure of the atriotomy. As a final maneuver, the air is evacuated through the vent at the apex of the anterior ventricle and the needle hole in the ascending aorta prior to defibrillation of the heart (*G*).

PLATE 105

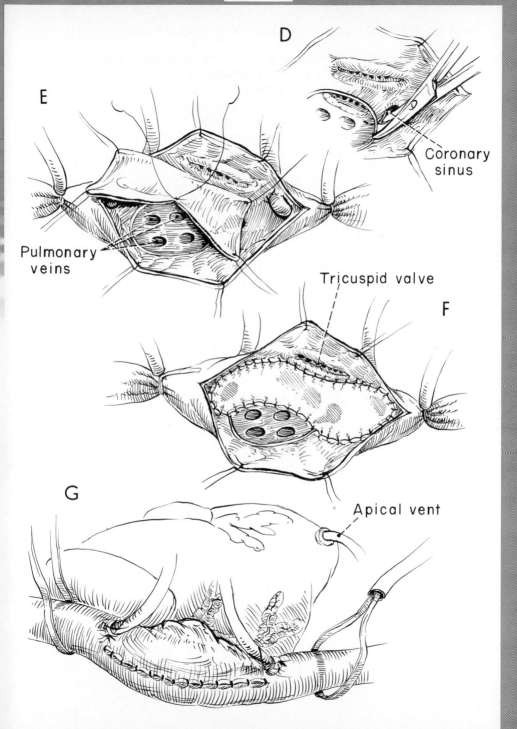

D

E

Coronary
sinus

Pulmonary
veins

Tricuspid valve

F

G

Apical vent

Left ventricular outflow tract obstruction may occur at various levels. In order of frequency, valvular, subvalvular and supravalvular obstructions can be enumerated. The most difficult to correct and, fortunately, the least common anomaly, is a combination of valvular and supravalvular malformation.

Subvalvular stenosis caused by a fibrous diaphragm below a normal valve provides an opportunity for an excellent operative result by simple excision of the fibrous ring.

Valvular stenosis may be an isolated lesion or may be associated with other conditions, such as coarctation of the aorta or hypoplasia of the left ventricle. If seen in childhood before secondary changes occur, the majority show three cusps which have failed to separate at their commissures. The leaflets may be quite equal in size (*B*) but more often are asymmetric even to the point of complete absence of one. The resulting bicuspid valve may or may not show some vestige of the third commissure (*A*).

Aortic valvotomy under direct vision can be performed through a median sternotomy incision. Cardiopulmonary by-pass is established and the aorta is clamped proximal to the innominate artery. The aortic valve is exposed through a longitudinal incision on the anterior wall of the aorta (*C*). Coronary perfusion is not necessary, since the procedure can be accomplished rapidly. The fused commissures are incised to the annulus, leaving the leaflets fused at this level (*D*). No attempt is made to incise a rudimentary commissure for fear of producing a severe aortic regurgitation. Closure is shown in *E*.

Supravalvular stenosis can be treated by the use of an oval-shaped Teflon patch (*F*) or by excision of the coarcted segment and end-to-end anastomosis (*G*), depending on the anatomy and the location of the constricted segment.

Degenerative changes, including severe degrees of calcification, preclude a satisfactory simple commissurotomy. Similarly, the anomalous valve may lack adequate commissural support elements. Everything must be in readiness for a valve replacement because of these possibilities.

PLATE 106

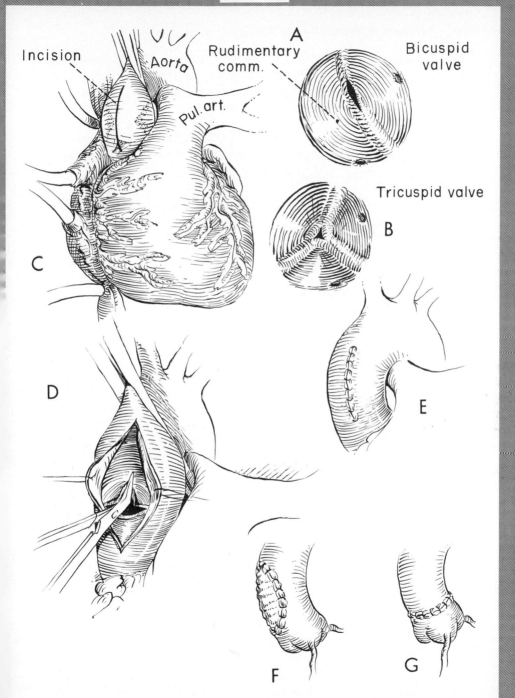

Incision
Aorta
Rudimentary comm.
Bicuspid valve
Pul. art.
A
Tricuspid valve
B
C
D
E
F
G

In the past several years there have been reports of a variety of surgical methods for relieving subaortic muscular hypertrophic stenosis. To expose the lesion, essentially two different approaches have been utilized: left ventriculotomy, with or without aortotomy, and left atriotomy with incision and retraction of the septal leaflet of the mitral valve. Regardless of the method of exposure, the goal is adequate resection of obstructive muscular and fibrotic tissues in the left ventricular outflow tract.

LEFT VENTRICULOTOMY APPROACH

The heart is exposed through a generous left anterolateral thoracotomy in the fifth intercostal space extending across the sternum (*A*). Preparations are then made for total cardiopulmonary by-pass. Cannulation of the right atrium via the atrial appendage and of the inferior vena cava retrograde via the common femoral vein eliminates the need for extending the thoracotomy into the right chest. After the institution of total by-pass, the apex of the heart is elevated into the wound and an incision about 1 in. long is made through the thin portion of the apex of the left ventricle. Digital palpation of the interior of the left ventricle serves to explore the lesion and at the same time to discover the optimum line of ventriculotomy. The incision is then extended anteriorly upward at least 1 cm. away from the anterior descending coronary artery. The upper limit of this incision depends on the position of the last major branch of the coronary artery. The posterior extension of the incision is virtually unlimited (*B*). This incision affords excellent exposure to the area of outflow obstruction and the mitral valve; the aortic valve is poorly visualized at first (*C*). In *D*, the general area of resection is shown, in which the aortic valve has come into full view. Closure of the ventriculotomy is accomplished with interrupted mattress sutures passed through a strip of Teflon along each margin of the incision. This is reinforced by a continuous over-and-over suture of nonabsorbable material.

[Left atriotomy approach *on page 330.*]

PLATE 109

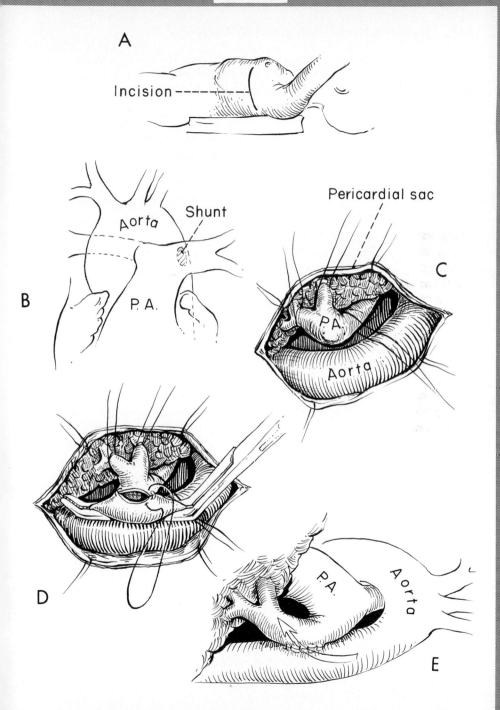

A

Incision ----

B

Aorta   Shunt

P.A.

Pericardial sac

C

P.A.

Aorta

D

P.A.   Aorta

E

Valvular pulmonic stenosis can be relieved by incising the valve with a valvulotome introduced through the right ventricular wall. This method is limited to isolated valvular pulmonic stenosis. It is effective in reducing, but does not always abolish, the difference in systolic pressures in the right ventricle and pulmonary artery. It is particularly useful in infants and small children when an emergency results from intractable heart failure secondary to the valvular stenosis.

Thoracotomy is through an anterolateral fifth intercostal space incision (*A*) or a vertical midline sternotomy. The approach illustrated is through the left chest. The fifth interspace incision is carried to the sternal edge and the pericardium opened (*B*).

A site in the outflow tract of the right ventricle is selected, sufficiently far from the valve ring that the valvulotome can be manipulated within the chamber without difficulty. This point is marked with a superficially placed pursestring suture (*C*).

A valvulotome of the type designed by Dr. Willis Potts is then introduced through the right ventricular wall with blades retracted (*D*) and is passed up into the pulmonary artery. The orifice of the stenotic valve may be so small as to be almost entirely occluded by the instrument. The blades are then opened (*E*) and, upon withdrawing the instrument into the ventricular cavity, the cutting edges on the proximal side incise the valve cone. This valvulotome is also available with blades on the forward edges of the expanded portion. After the valvulotome is removed, further disruption of the stenosis can be accomplished by placing in the orifice an expandable dilator, also designed by Potts.

PLATE 110

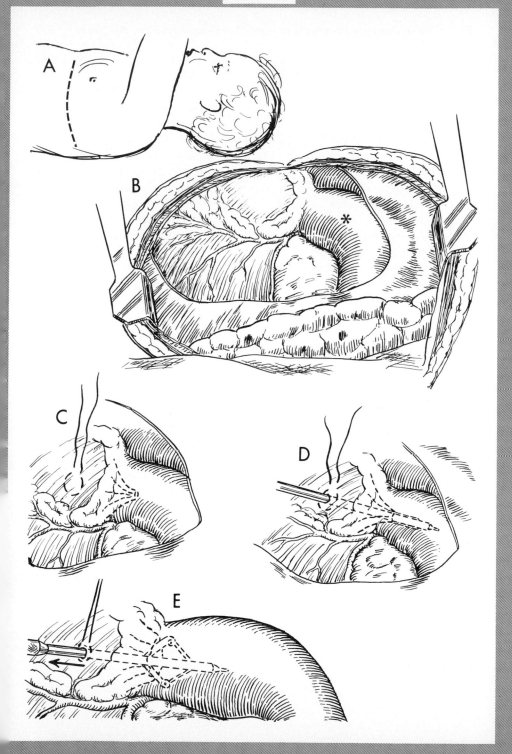

More advanced techniques in the relief of valvular pulmonic stenosis of the congenital type have essentially replaced transventricular valvulotomy except as an emergency procedure in infants in heart failure. The more advanced techniques include (1) hypothermia and inflow occlusion and (2) cardiopulmonary by-pass using the pump-oxygenator. Both permit direct exposure of the valve through an incision in the pulmonary artery. The time available for actual work on the valve using hypothermia is entirely adequate to achieve complete relief of the valvular stenosis. It is inadequate for repair in the presence of a hypoplasia of the pulmonary valve ring or of significant subvalvular outflow tract obstruction either of congenital origin or acquired by work hypertrophy of the muscle.

Pulmonary valvulotomy during extracorporeal circulation is done through a sternum-splitting incision. The pump connections are made and the pulmonary artery isolated and obstructed as far as possible from the valve ring (*A*). Figures *B–D*, detailing the exposure through the pulmonary artery, are viewed from the position of the surgeon on the right of the patient. A longitudinal incision is made in the pulmonary artery, exposing a typical cone-shaped, fibrous valve structure (*B*), in which there is little if any indication of normal commissural architecture.

This cone is usually much elongated and, therefore, in addition to incisions which extend all the way to the valve ring, the tip is amputated as indicated in *C*. A bivalve structure is thus produced (*D*), and the stenosis is completely relieved unless there is some degree of valve ring hypoplasia. A degree of pulmonary regurgitation sufficient to produce a murmur often results without clinical evidence of a significant hemodynamic defect.

PLATE 111

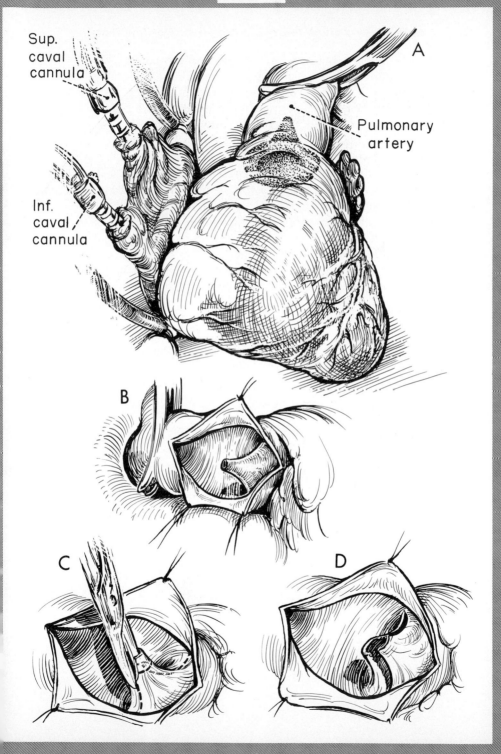

Sup.
caval
cannula

Pulmonary
artery

Inf.
caval
cannula

A

B

C

D

Complete relief of resistance in the pulmonary outflow tract and the pulmonary valve may not be obtained in isolated valvular pulmonic stenosis by simple pulmonary valvulotomy. Enlargement of the outflow tract of the right ventricle may also be required when there is either an atresia of the pulmonary valve ring (*A*) or a severe muscular hypertrophy of the outflow tract (*D*) which has resulted from a long-standing congenital stenosis of the pulmonary valve.

The valve ring must be enlarged when it is underdeveloped. This situation is recognized after the pulmonary artery has been opened for incision of the stenosed valve. The pulmonary arteriotomy is then extended down through the ring for a distance of 3 – 4 cm. into the infundibular channel (*B*). The valve is incised in that point of its circumference coinciding to the incision in the valve ring, and the orifice may be further enlarged by an incision in the remaining portion of the cone directly opposite. The entire incision is then repaired using a teardrop-shaped patch of woven Dacron or Teflon, as shown in *C*. This obviously results in an incompetence of the pulmonary valve which is apparently well tolerated.

There may be sufficient hypertrophy of the right ventricular wall in relation to the outflow channel (*D*) to obstruct the passage of the operator's fifth finger down through the incised valve into the heart. It is likely that this muscular hypertrophy would reverse itself after removal of the obstruction, but free outflow from the right ventricle can be obtained immediately by enlarging the area with a prosthetic patch. An incision is made in the outflow tract of the right ventricle from a point proximal to the valve ring downward for 3 – 5 cm. (*E*). This incision is closed using a patch (*F*). The teardrop shape of the patch seems to have an architectural advantage over an ellipse.

F also indicates that the longitudinal wound in the pulmonary artery is simply closed in a routine manner without the addition of an enlarging prosthesis.

PLATE 112

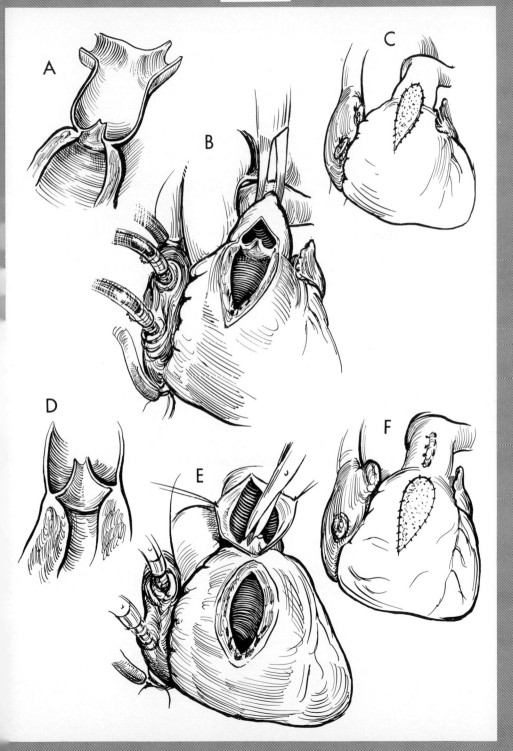

Tetralogy of Fallot is a complex congenital malformation composed of a large ventricular septal defect, pulmonary stenosis of sufficient severity to cause a right-to-left shunt, dextraposition of the aorta and right ventricular hypertrophy. The object of surgical management is to abolish pulmonary stenosis by removal of the infundibular muscle mass in addition to pulmonary valvotomy if indicated, and to close the awkwardly situated ventricular septal defect without producing atrioventricular block.

The presence of severe hypoplastic pulmonary arteries contraindicates surgical intervention for total correction. In these infants a systemic pulmonary shunt should be considered first, in the hope that gradual enlargement of the pulmonary arteries will take place, preparing the lesion for a complete repair at a later stage.

A median sternotomy provides the best exposure (*A*). The pericardium is incised longitudinally and cannulation is effected. The left ventricle is vented through an apical stab wound. After total by-pass has begun, the aorta is cross-clamped. The right ventricular incision is positioned in such a manner as to avoid major branches of the right coronary artery. The incision may therefore vary from a vertical (*B*) to a transverse direction. The obstruction to the outflow tract is often caused by the thickened wall of the right ventricle and abnormally situated crista supraventricularis. Excision of a layer of muscle in the infundibular portion (*C*), in addition to undercutting to separate the ventricular wall from the crista, provides adequate passage for pulmonary flow. The pulmonary valve should be examined and incised in two directions if necessary (*D*).

The exposure of the ventricular septal defect is improved by the infundibular resection. A patch of Dacron graft is uniformly needed for the repair of this high-lying and poorly circumscribed defect. Interrupted and transversely placed sutures on the right ventricular side of the defect along the inferoposterior margin avoids the conduction bundle (*E*). The ventriculotomy is then closed with a double row of continuous sutures, approximating the superficial layer of the myocardial wall (*F*). Air is evacuated through the right ventriculotomy suture line, left ventricular vent and needle puncture at the root of the aorta.

PLATE 113

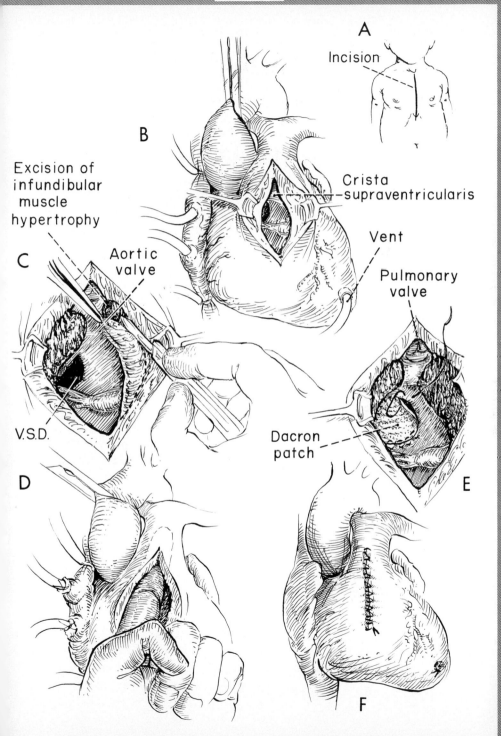

A

Incision

B

Excision of
infundibular
muscle
hypertrophy

Crista
supraventricularis

Vent

Aortic
valve

Pulmonary
valve

C

V.S.D.

Dacron
patch

D

E

F

CHAPTER 24

Heart Transplantation

THE PATIENT with end-stage heart disease for whom no other treatment is available is a candidate for cardiac transplantation. The procedure involves a recipient and a donor and, therefore, requires two operative teams in adjacent operating rooms, each with monitoring systems and facilities for cardiopulmonary by-pass.

The recipient is moved to the operating room at a time estimated to coincide with the anticipated death of the donor. It may be advisable to postpone general anesthesia until preparations have been made for partial by-pass under local anesthesia using the common femoral vessels (*A*). Retrograde cannulation of the inferior vena cava facilitates implantation. The superior vena cava is cannulated through a stab wound in the right atrial wall near the atrial caval junction. The aorta and pulmonary artery are encircled with cord tapes. Upon institution of total by-pass at normothermia, vascular clamps are placed across the distal ascending aorta and the pulmonary artery. With the superior and inferior venae cavae occluded, the heart is excised, leaving most of the right and left atria, the atrial septum, the proximal aorta and pulmonary artery (*B*).

The donor's heart is exposed through a median sternotomy. Dissection is carried out to encircle the aorta, pulmonary artery, the right pulmonary veins and the venae cavae. The superior vena cava is ligated at the atrial caval junction. In this way the implanted organ will retain its entire autonomic nervous system (*C*).

The recipient is placed on total by-pass and the heart excised as described. The donor's entire heart is then removed. The left atrium is incised posteriorly (*C*). Under ideal circumstances it is feasible to implant the organ without coronary perfusion. In most

PLATE 114

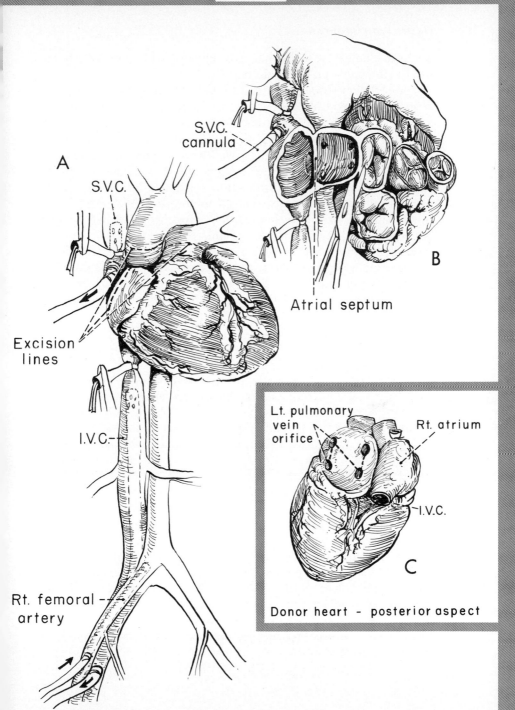

A

S.V.C.

Excision
lines

I.V.C.

Rt. femoral
artery

S.V.C.
cannula

Atrial septum

B

Lt. pulmonary
vein orifice

Rt. atrium

I.V.C.

C

Donor heart – posterior aspect

instances, however, maintenance of myocardial oxygenization during the implantation is mandatory.

The technique of suturing can be carried out with the following sequential steps. First the left atrial connection is made with the attachment of the medial border of the donor's left atrial opening to the recipient's septum. Then the right atrial opening, which had been made by incising the atrial wall from the inferior vena caval orifice to the base of the atrial appendage, is anastomosed to the recipient's right atrium. Once again the posterior border of the right atrial opening is anastomosed to the recipient's septum. In this manner the entire septum of the donor's heart, which actually is not seen during implantation, is preserved.

The pulmonary and aortic anastomoses are done next. Release of the aortic clamp results in retrograde perfusion of the coronary arteries and permits removal of air from the left side of the heart. The heart begins to fibrillate, and it is possible that it might spontaneously revert into contractions or need an electric shock to interrupt the ventricular fibrillation.

If coronary arteries are perfused, the following technique of suturing is employed. The left atrial anastomosis is done first (D). This is followed by pulmonary artery anastomosis. The aortic anastomosis is then completed except for a small opening to permit the coronary catheters to remain in place. At this time the right atrium is incised from the inferior vena caval orifice to the base of the atrial appendage, and this opening is anastomosed to the recipient's right atrium (E). At this time the oxygenated coronary sinus blood returning from the lungs permits filling of the left heart chambers with blood and evacuation of air. Venting of the left ventricle will not be necessary. The coronary catheters are removed as the remaining part of the aortic anastomosis is closed (F), permitting release of the aortic clamp to maintain coronary perfusion.

The air is removed from the ascending aorta either by releasing the aortic clamp before completing closure of the aortotomy or by making one or two needle holes in the anterior aspect of the ascending aorta. The cannulas are removed, protamine sulfate is given to neutralize heparin and the patient is placed in an isolated room where sterile precautions are maintained and physiologic functions are monitored.

PLATE 114

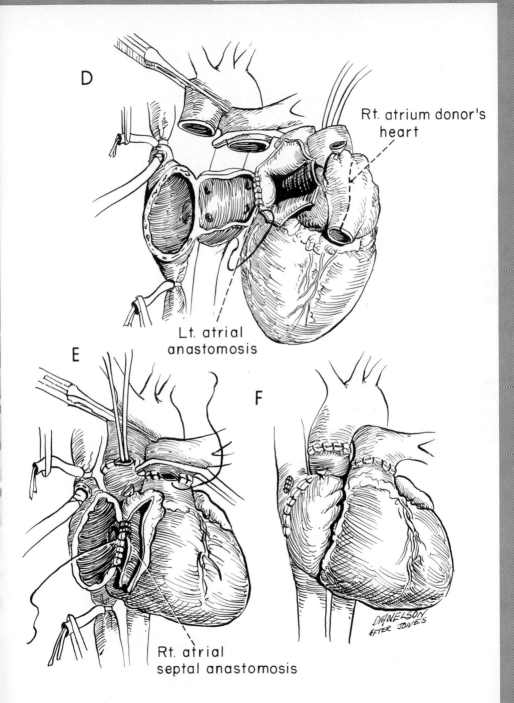

D

Rt. atrium donor's heart

Lt. atrial anastomosis

E

F

Rt. atrial septal anastomosis

DANELSON AFTER JONES

CHAPTER **25**

Cardiac Resuscitation

THE SIGNS of cessation of circulation due to the loss of efficient cardiac action result from cardiac arrest in diastole, ventricular fibrillation and depression of cardiac contractions to such a low level that cardiac action is undetectable. This last situation of reduced cardiac output seems important, because it is as strong an indication for resuscitative treatment as cardiac arrest in diastole or ventricular fibrillation. If the low output is allowed to persist, cardiac arrest by the other mechanisms will occur. Under all these circumstances, circulation and respiration must be supported artificially while measures are taken to restore cardiac action and to correct the cause of the incident, if it can be determined.

Not all patients who suffer circulatory collapse are candidates for cardiac resuscitation. This issue is confused, because in an emergency the patient's background is not always known to the one who must decide immediately as to treatment. Fundamentally, the indication to start resuscitation or to continue it may be said to depend on whether the underlying problem is correctible. Thus, cardiac arrest would not be subject to treatment in a patient who has had chronic heart failure under good medical management, or who is known to have extensive and severe arteriosclerotic heart disease, or whose cardiac arrest is an expression of the termination of an illness such as carcinoma or renal failure.

The extent and complexity of the resuscitative measures needed vary with the cause of the event. A simple physical stimulus may restore cardiac action in a patient with a Stokes-Adams attack, whereas all types of treatment may have to be used before success is attained in a patient with ventricular fibrillation. The environment in which the problem is met has little bearing on the indication for treatment, although it indirectly determines the proportion of the causes of arrest which are met. Thus, ventricular fibrillation following a coronary occlusion which would not in itself cause fatal myocardial damage would be one of the most frequent causes in a nonmedical environment in which hope of success would justify the use of resuscitation. In a doctor's office, in an x-ray department or in the dental chair the emergency may occur in response to an injection or to the topical application of some drug. In the operating room, contributing causes will be the anesthetic agents, anoxia or blood loss.

The locale of occurrence has, however, a marked effect on the chances of success of resuscitation. The availability of assistance, of equipment and of transport to a medical facility has a strong bearing. Little can be said in regard to an individual physician's responsibility to initiate treatment in the wide variety of situations, except that a readiness in the way of some equipment and, certainly, of information is expected in areas under his control, such as his office. Hospitals, on the other hand, must accept the expense and responsibility of having every element of equipment needed and of keeping it available and in good working condition.

The basic steps in resuscitation are (1) immediate diagnosis, (2) provision of an effective cardiac output by mechanical means, (3) provision of adequate respiration through a clear airway, (4) correction of the cause, (5) observation of the patient for recurrence of arrest and (6) support of the patient in regard to any damage he may have sustained during the anoxic period of the arrest.

Immediacy of diagnosis must be stressed because of the brain damage produced by more than a few minutes of severe anoxia. The emergency is sufficiently dramatic that, when it occurs under observation, the only differential diagnosis is that of other causes of loss of consciousness. The combination of loss of consciousness and complete loss of pulses in the femoral and carotid regions is diagnostic of low cardiac output collapse. Differentiation from suffocation, such as that due to aspiration of a foreign body into the trachea, can hardly be a problem if the episode occurs under observation.

Diagnosis in the operating room is much more direct. The lack of pulsation in a major vessel during abdominal or extremity surgery or the observed cardiac action during an intrathoracic procedure supplements the continuous watchfulness of the anesthetist in diagnosis. An effective cardiac output is obtained by direct manual compression of the heart if the chest is open, by compression of the heart through the diaphragm or trans-sternally through the closed chest if the abdomen is open and by trans-sternal compression of the heart under all other circumstances.

The demonstration by Jude and Kouwenhoven that compression of the heart by pressure on the sternum results in an effective circulation has entirely changed the practical and emotional approach to this problem. This method should be applied without recourse to thoracotomy for direct manual systole as long as it is demonstrated to be effective. The technique is given in Plate 115.

As external manual systole is instituted, the airway is cleared and, through successive stages of refinement, controlled respiration is established. Oronasal insufflation of the lungs may be followed by insufflation through an oral airway, and finally endotracheal intubation allows for connection to an anesthesia machine for positive insufflation of the lungs. Now follows a period in which the circulation and respiration are under control, permitting consideration of measures to correct the cause of the emergency. From a general standpoint, the frequent cause, anoxia, will have been remedied by the positive respiratory exchange. Blood loss, which may have been a cause or an important contributing factor if the incident occurs during surgery, is now replaced. As these general measures of correction are going on, preparations are made for diagnosing the type of abnormality in cardiac action by means of electrocardiograph. An electrocardiogram may define the difficulty as one of slow, ineffective heart rate, ventricular fibrillation or total asystole. The support of the circulation manually and correction of the cause will often be sufficient to restore cardiac action in patients in whom it has not actually entirely ceased or in patients arrested in diastole. Ventricular fibrillation, if present, must be corrected through the application of an externally applied electric shock (Plate 115). If manual systole is being applied directly to the heart because the cardiac arrest occurred during a thoracic operation or because external compression failed to produce adequate circulation, the electric shock is applied directly to the surface of the heart. Suitable external and internal defibrillators are available as separate or combined units and are a necessary part of hospital equipment for cardiac resuscitation.

Cardiac-stimulating drugs may help restore ventricular contractions when arrest in diastole is present. Calcium ions in the form of calcium chloride solution given in doses of 0.5 – 1 Gm. intravenously are also useful. When cardiac action consists of a slow, ineffective contraction, Isuprel in small doses intravenously (0.05 mg.) is given, as well as epinephrine and calcium. Calcium and small doses of epinephrine may also be useful in ventricular fibrillation if the fibrillatory activity is weak and the first application of an electric shock fails to convert it. Isuprel is damaging in ventricular fibrillation. A critical period follows the restoration of regular ventricular contractions, during which time recurrence of arrest may occur. The team must remain in readiness to support weakening contractions by addition of manual compression before the diminishing output culminates in further myocardial anoxia, which in itself depresses the cardiac action. If a period of manual systole has been prolonged, the patient should empirically be considered to be in acidosis of the metabolic type, likely well compensated by excessive removal of carbon dioxide by the efficient mechanically supported respirations. The intravenous administration of sodium bicarbonate in a few repeated doses of 30 – 50 mEq. will support cardiac action because it will partially overcome the acidosis.

If there was delay in starting resuscitation, or if a significant degree of partial anoxia existed during a long period of treatment, brain damage may be evident immediately and its signs deepen progressively after cardiac action has been restored. A significant factor in brain damage is the edema which develops after a period of anoxia. The extent of the edema is diminished by placing the patient under prolonged moderate hypothermia, using a heat exchange blanket or applying ice bags externally. An additional measure in combating cerebral edema is the intravenous administration of urea.

CLOSED-CHEST CARDIAC COMPRESSION

The patient is placed on his back on a firm surface for cardiac compression to begin while every arrangement is being made for the maintenance of controlled respiration. The patient may well be placed on the floor, where the operator can kneel at either side and position himself with his own shoulders over the patient's lower sternum, his arms extended and his hands placed flat, one on top of the other, on the middle and lower portions of the sternum (*A*). Force is then applied to the sternum rhythmically at a rate of 70–80 times per minute. Maximum force is not used; rather, sufficient force is applied to depress the sternum a distance corresponding to about 1½ in. in a young adult. Each compression is followed by complete relaxation of the sternum to allow for cardiac filling. It is essential that the efficiency of the cardiac compression be continuously monitored by the presence of a femoral artery pulse with each stroke. If a pulse is not produced, venous return to the heart may be improved by elevating the lower extremities, and a better compression may be obtained by increasing the force of the pressure or by shifting the point of its application.

The cross-section of the thorax in *B* indicates that the ventricular and atrioventricular areas of the heart are more or less efficiently compressed when the sternum is forcefully pushed toward the dorsal spine. The efficiency of external compression is diminished in emphysema with the increased anteroposterior diameter of the chest, in funnel deformity and by rigidity of the chest wall in some older patients.

EXTERNAL DEFIBRILLATION

The broad electrodes of the external defibrillator are applied over the chest in the midventricular and apical region for one point and the upper sternal area for the second (*C*). These electrodes are applied quickly and firmly as the hands of the person applying external compression are completely withdrawn. The handles of the equipment are arranged in a manner such that the person holding the two electrodes cannot come into contact with the electric current, but care must be taken not to give an electric shock to others working about the patient.

PLATE 115

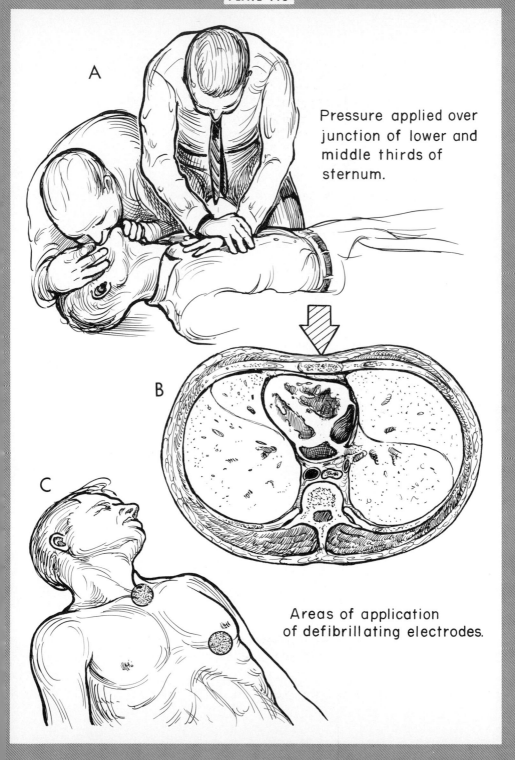

A

Pressure applied over junction of lower and middle thirds of sternum.

B

C

Areas of application of defibrillating electrodes.

Index

353